The Double Fat-Burning Exercise Program

The Double Fat-Burning *Exercise* Program

Paul Galbraith D.C.

A LOTHIAN BOOK

Acknowledgements

Felicia, Byron, Tasha – for putting up with me while I was writing this book.
Jacqui – for typing and trying to read my writing.

A Lothian Book
Thomas C. Lothian Pty Ltd
11 Munro Street, Port Melbourne, Victoria 3207

Copyright © Paul Galbraith 1995
First published 1995

All rights reserved. No part of this publication may be reproduced, stored in a retrieval system or transmitted in any form by any means without the prior permission of the copyright owner.
Enquiries should be made to the publisher.

National Library of Australia
Cataloguing-in-Publication data:

Galbraith, Paul, 1947-
The double fat-burning exercise program.

Bibliography
Includes index.
ISBN 0 85091 683 6

1. Reducing exercises. 2. Physical fitness.
I. Title.
567.91

Text design and illustrations by Lynn Twelftree
Cover design by David Constable
Photographs by Con Macarlino

Typeset by Image Makers, South Melbourne, in Utopia 11 pt
Printed in Australia by Griffin Paperbacks

Contents

Introduction 6

Part 1 • The Secret to Permanent Fat Loss
Good Reasons to Become Slim 10
The Basic Problem and Five Myths About Slimming 12
Why Diets Always Fail 18
The Mental Aspect of Slimming 25
Successful Slimming for Females 34
Common Questions About Weight Control 36

Part 2 • The Double Fat-burning Exercise Program
How the Double Fat-burning Exercise Program Works 40
How to Exercise Correctly 49
The Double Fat-burning Exercises 55
The Five-minute Super Fat Loss Exercises 61

Part 3 • Eat Yourself Thin—The Nutritional Approach
The Nutritional Way to Quick and Permanent Fat Loss 74
It's What and When You Eat That's Important 94
Ten Foods to Help You Slim 96
Tips for Losing Fat Quickly and Keeping It Off 98
Fifty Painless Ways to Cut Kilojoules 105

Part 4 • Looking Even Better
Trimming Your Thighs 112
The Most Potent Exercises to Firm Your Hips and Buttocks 118
How to Shed Your Potbelly 120

Putting it Together 129

Recipes to Help You Stay Slim 131

Further Reading 159

Index 160

Introduction

Why do we become fat? The main reason is the fact that as we get older our metabolic rate slows down. This slow-down usually begins at about twenty-seven years of age and continues at a rate of five per cent every ten years. It means that your body burns fewer kilojoules and therefore *more* kilojoules are stored as fat on the body. And, because body fat burns fewer kilojoules than lean muscle tissue does, overweight people easily become even more overweight.

The slowing down of the metabolic rate as we age is one of the natural physiological changes associated with ageing and is seen very plainly in everyday life. The majority of people who are overweight do not eat more food than when they were younger. In fact, many people eat less than they used to and still become fatter and are unable to lose the excess fat. The only thing that has changed is their metabolism, which has slowed down. The latest research shows that people who don't put on weight and eat a lot have a metabolic rate that is up to 35 per cent higher than average; that is, they use 35 per cent more energy just to exist.

So, our metabolic rate slows down as we age—that's the bad news. The good news is that this rate can be speeded up and remain at a higher level all day by doing the right type of exercise. I stress the *right* type of exercise because experience shows that most people who exercise are not exercising properly and do not achieve maximum fat loss and optimum fitness. Often, people do more harm than good by exercising incorrectly.

It's been known for some time that correctly performed aerobic exercise, such as jogging, brisk walking and aerobics increases the metabolic rate, but recently it's been discovered that muscle-stimulating exercises also increase the metabolic rate. Obviously, the ideal exercise system is one where the exercises are both aerobic and muscle-stimulating at the same time. This means you are achieving a double increase of your metabolic rate and therefore a double fat-burning effect, and no extra time is required. This is the optimum exercise program for losing maximum fat in the shortest possible time.

This book describes in detail, with photographs, the best exercises to do. You are shown how to obtain the maximum aerobic effect from the exercises and which exercises are both aerobic and muscle-stimulating.

Also, when you perform exercises which are aerobic, it's very important to exercise for the correct duration and extremely important to exercise at the correct intensity. If you exercise below the correct intensity level, you will not achieve maximum fat loss and if you exercise above the correct intensity level you will adversely effect your health. You are shown how to calculate accurately the correct exercise intensity for your age using a formula. Alternatively, you may look at the chart (on page 52) and see what your ideal exercise intensity is for your age.

Diets Don't Work

Science and experience verify this. Unfortunately, diets do nothing to solve the basic problem of a slower metabolic rate. On the contrary, research shows that diets actually slow down the metabolic rate. Experience also proves this; most people who diet actually put on more weight after they finish dieting. The chapter called 'Why Diets Always Fail', explains the reasons for this in detail.

Australians are fat; very fat according to the latest National Heart Foundation summary of the nation's health. This showed that a massive 42 per cent of people over thirty-five years of age are overweight or obese. Furthermore, one-quarter to one-third of under 16s also fit into this category. The situation in the USA is even worse.

The average person is likely to carry far more fat compared with twenty years ago but this trend has been partly hidden by clothing manufacturers. According to a recent *Bulletin* survey, the average woman's dress size has increased a size and a half over the past twenty years. Cunningly, manufacturers have kept to the old sizes while increasing the measurements. Thus a size twelve, the average size which used to fit an 85-centimetre waist and 95.5-centimetre hip, is now six centimetres bigger at the waist and hip.

Frequently, people who are overweight will tell you they do plenty of exercise and don't overeat. They can't understand why they can't lose weight. These people may be doing a lot of exercise but you can almost guarantee they are doing the wrong type of exercise or doing it the wrong way—at least for the purpose of losing fat. Housework is often very hard work and physically tiring but, you see, this is not the optimum type of exercise for losing fat. Even people doing hard manual labour are usually not doing the best type of exercise for losing fat.

Similarly, for those people who know they don't overeat but still can't lose weight, you can bet that most of them are eating the wrong type of foods.

By following the exercise program in this book you will become slimmer and also attain a higher level of fitness. This means your body will function better—including your brain, nerves, glands and internal organs.

You will have more vitality all day and sleep deeply at night. You will be less likely to develop a serious illness such as heart disease, high blood pressure, cancer or diabetes. In addition, you will look younger and your muscles will become healthier and firmer, including your facial muscles which will achieve a natural face lift. Women will develop firmer breast muscles and sagging breasts will be given a natural lift. Men and women will develop a more powerful chest which affects not only appearance but also increases the health of the two organs within the chest—the heart and lungs.

As you can see, there is a lot to gain besides just losing fat. Just start the program and the results will ensure you keep going. Since this program is not severe—you don't have to give up all your favourite foods or exercise strenuously—and because your health and vitality will improve, you would be wise to make this a *lifetime* program.

Part One

The Secret to Permanent Fat Loss

Good Reasons to Become Slim

FIRST—HOW TO TELL IF YOU ARE OVERWEIGHT

There are three easy ways to tell if you are overweight. These are:

The Mirror Test

Just take your clothes off and stand in front of the mirror. Can you see any extra flesh where there shouldn't be? Remember, the mirror doesn't lie.

The Pinch Test

Pinch a good layer of skin over your tummy. If you can pinch more than 2.5 centimetres you're likely to benefit from losing some body fat.

Waist to Hip Ratio

Measure your waist and hips. Divide your waist measurement by your hip measurement. A number bigger than 0.95 for men and 0.85 for women is too high.

THE EFFECTS OF BEING OVERWEIGHT

While most people go on diets purely for cosmetic reasons, to look and feel more attractive, there are strong medical reasons for reducing weight. If you are just slightly overweight, you will feel unfit and a little tired.

However, once a person reaches a weight of 10 per cent or more above the ideal, then serious effects start to appear.

The Physical Risks

An overweight person is more likely to suffer from illness and has a greater risk of dying young than someone of normal weight. The further you are from your ideal weight, the greater the risk, particularly for people who are overweight before the age of thirty-five.

The more overweight you are, the higher your chances of suffering from problems with blood pressure, diabetes, back trouble, respiratory infections and hardening of the arteries of the heart (which can lead to stroke and heart attacks) gallstones, bronchitis and varicose veins. Bones and joints also take a greater strain when you are obese and this can lead to other problems. Fat people are more prone to accidents as they often find it more difficult to move quickly.

Physical exertion is generally difficult for many obese people and consequently their lifestyle is often more restricted compared with other people. Fatness stops you from being fit; you become breathless and strained with any effort. Surgeons find it more difficult to examine or operate on obese patients and important signs of disease may be overlooked. There is also a danger of post-operative complications.

The Psychological Effects

These can be as bad as the physical effects of fatness and obesity and can severely hamper efforts to lose weight and stay slim. Being overweight can lead to feelings of inadequacy and depression, can destroy self-confidence and self-esteem. The overweight person also has to deal with the emotional pressures of a society which looks on slimness as the ideal form.

The Basic Problem and Five Myths about Slimming

When your body is carrying excess fat it is not in a natural state. A few generations ago fatness wasn't a widespread problem; it seems that nowadays we are either doing or not doing things that were once part of daily life. If you examine carefully how we live now and how we used to live, you'll find there are two major differences. First, we do far less physical exercise than our ancestors and, second, we eat far more processed foods. This change in lifestyle is affecting the way our bodies work, and two of the results of this are disease and excess fat.

LACK OF CORRECT EXERCISE AND YOUR WEIGHT PROBLEM

The average person today has a very sedentary lifestyle. A lot of people sit in offices all day and even manual workers have machines to do the hard work. Instead of walking we tend to travel by car or bus, and in the home we have many labour-saving devices. Our ancestors had a totally different lifestyle, hunting wild animals and walking everywhere. In addition, there were no labour-saving devices in the living place.

Our bodies are not designed to run on processed foods and they are also not designed to be sedentary. As we get older our metabolic rate slows down and so our fat reserves are not burnt up as efficiently as when we were younger, resulting in a gradual accumulation of fat. If we did sustained physical exercise, as our ancestors did, this fat build-up would not occur. This is because sustained exercise for at least fifteen minutes, with a pulse rate of at least 75 per cent of our maximum possible rate, causes our metabolic rate to speed up. This type of exercise is called aerobic exercise. The exercise system described in this book combines aerobic exercises and muscle-stimulating exercises at the same time and is the fastest way to lose fat.

An increase in metabolic rate due to aerobic/muscle-stimulating exercises occurs not just during the exercise period, but for the whole day, even while you are sleeping. Your excess fat will be burnt up more quickly, resulting in a new, slimmer you. The sort of exercise you need to do is discussed in detail in Part 2, pages 40–72.

PROCESSED FOODS AND YOUR WEIGHT PROBLEM

What are Processed Foods?

Food processing can be described as altering in some way the natural state of fresh food. Processed foods have usually been heated and/or chemicals added to them. They are usually high in fat and sugar and therefore a major cause of weight gain, health problems and premature ageing.

Unfortunately most of the foods you buy in supermarkets are processed and therefore you should try to be very selective.

Processed foods have had most of their nutritional value destroyed, and are loaded with harmful chemicals. In addition, because processing removes most of the fibre from the food, the foods are low in bulk and this often results in colon problems, such as constipation, and a predisposition to cancer of the bowel.

The chemicals added to food include preservatives, colourings, flavourings and texturisers. Preservatives allow a vast range of modern foodstuffs to be available all year round on the shop shelves. Preservatives are used to stop food from being spoiled by the growth of bacteria and fungi, to prevent natural processes within the food from making it inedible, and to prevent the process of oxidation. Colourings are added to make food look more attractive, since a lot of food when processed loses its natural colour. Flavourings include chemicals like salt and MSG (monosodium glutamate). MSG is actually flavourless but has the property of enhancing flavour in meat and fish products. Since its discovery in 1908, it has been used increasingly by food manufacturers, and is used in many Asian dishes. A small proportion of people are actually allergic to MSG and it should be avoided by asthma sufferers. Texturisers are used in foods like ice-cream to give it that characteristic creamy texture.

More than 3000 different chemicals are now used in processed foods. Very little is known about some of these chemicals and their long-term effects. Appetite stimulants are particularly bad since they lead to overeating and, even worse, the overeating of junk food. This sort of diet results in poor nourishment, obesity and ultimately disease and premature ageing.

Appetite stimulants, such as salt and spices, also cause the taste buds of the tongue to lose their sensitivity. This leads to an addiction to processed foods and the inability to enjoy the subtle flavours of simple natural foods.

The heating of food destroys the enzymes or the life-promoting part of the food. Enzymes speed up chemical reactions in the body up to several thousandfold and therefore without them we could not survive—they are even more important than vitamins. Heat-treating food gives it a longer shelf life since no self-respecting weevil or other bug would want to eat it—a weevil knows by instinct there is very little nutrition in processed food.

How Processed Foods Cause Weight Problems

Eating processed foods causes an increase in weight in three ways. First, these foods usually have a high fat and sugar content. Second, they are usually low in nutrients. This means your body must take in more food in an attempt to obtain an adequate nutrient intake. Your body does this by maintaining an appetite to encourage you to eat more. The body's instinct for survival overrides any conscious attempt to lose weight. Third, many processed foods contain chemicals called appetisers. These chemicals increase your appetite, causing you to overeat and put on even more weight.

If you think about it, only processed foods have a high fat and sugar content. For example butter, cheese, margarine, vegetable oils, chocolate, ice-cream, cakes, pizzas and so on are all processed foods. Butter does not come from a cow. The milk from the cow is processed and concentrated, so you are just eating the fat from the milk.

As you can see, processed foods are a major cause of excess fat build-up.

The Solution

Try to reduce the amount of processed food you eat, replacing it with fresh foods such as fruit, vegetables and unrefined grain products.

Replace white bread with wholemeal bread, preferably made with stoneground wholemeal flour; this is readily available in supermarkets (e.g. Vogel's wholemeal and sesame seed bread).

Reduce the amount of canned food you eat. Canned food is heated to very high temperatures which destroys most of the vitamins and minerals and 100 per cent of the enzymes. The manufacturers' intention is to destroy all the enzymes, since then the food is 'dead' and will keep for long periods.

Don't peel your potatoes, since the peel contains most of a potato's nutrients. Cook potatoes in their jackets. When cooking, replace salt, pepper and spices such as MSG with natural nutritious flavours from garlic, onions, herbs and lemon juice.

In short, our bodies have not evolved to cope with the lifestyle we now live. Our physiological and biochemical mechanisms are designed to metabolise natural fresh foods, not processed foods, and to live a physically active life. The majority of people have a diet which mainly consists of processed foods and do no exercise or not the correct type of exercise. These two factors would account for at least 90 per cent of our diseases, minor ailments and premature ageing. In addition, of course, we become fat.

The rest of this book will show you how to make the change, that is, to get the maximum effect from the right exercise and the right food. You will not only lose fat, but you will also feel better and look younger.

Five Myths About Slimming

Myth No. 1 ● *The Main Issue is Your Weight*

You actually need to lose fat but not necessarily weight. If you slim the correct way, as outlined in this book, you will lose fat but possibly no weight. You will certainly be much slimmer due to the fat loss. On the double fat-burning exercise program the fat that is lost is replaced by lean muscle and, since muscle weighs more than fat, there may be no overall weight loss. Dieters lose weight because they are losing healthy lean muscle as well as fat.

Most experts now suggest that you should throw away your bathroom scales and judge your fatness by your waist measurement and the tightness of your clothes.

Myth No. 2 ● *Calorie Counting is the Answer*

We are fatter today than we were fifty years ago yet we eat less than our recent ancestors. These historical statistics which come from food production figures through the years imply that there is more to the story than eating too many kilojoules.

The obvious explanation of this situation is energy expenditure. Our great-grandparents were much more active and they burned up more kilojoules doing incidental exercise, such as climbing stairs instead of catching a lift.

If small daily exercises have such an effect you can imagine how much more effective aerobic exercise is, where the activity is reasonably strenuous and for a sustained period of time. Because of the sedentary lifestyle we live today it is essential we do this type of exercise, both for fat control and health.

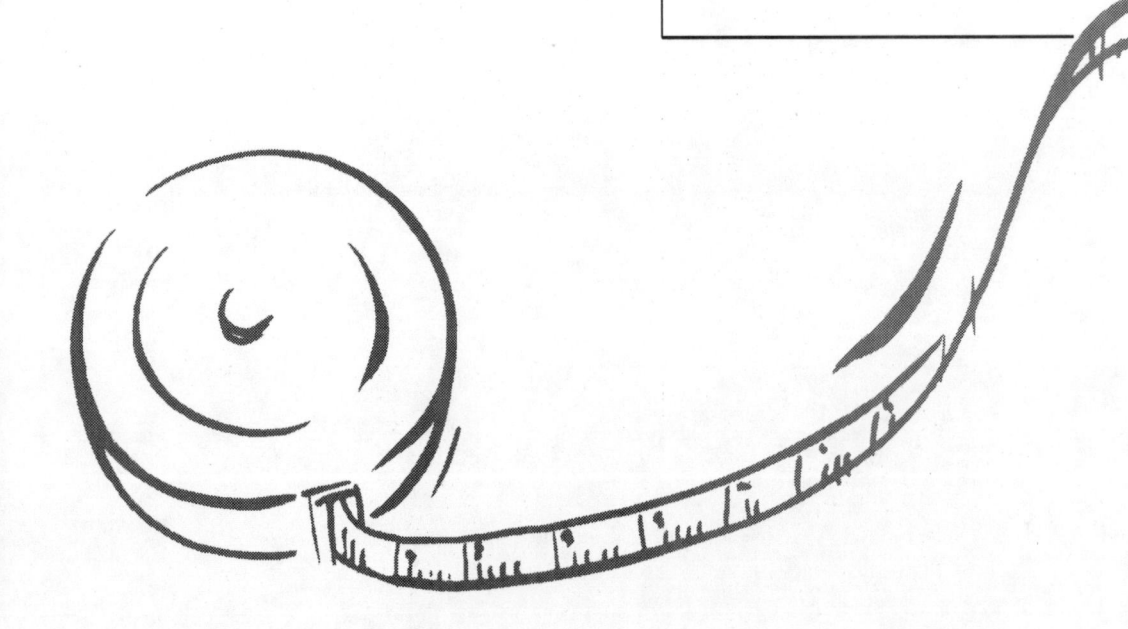

Myth No. 3 ● *Fat People Eat More than Thin People*

Studies actually show that thin people eat more than fat people. Again, this demonstrates that kilojoule reduction is not the main factor in losing fat. Thin people have higher metabolic rates than fat people because they have a higher muscle to fat ratio, and muscle has a higher metabolic rate than fat.

The only way fat people can get rid of their fat is by reducing their fat/sugar intake and doing aerobic/muscle-stimulating exercises. Once you lose your excess fat you reduce the possibility of becoming fat again, since you will have a slim person's metabolism.

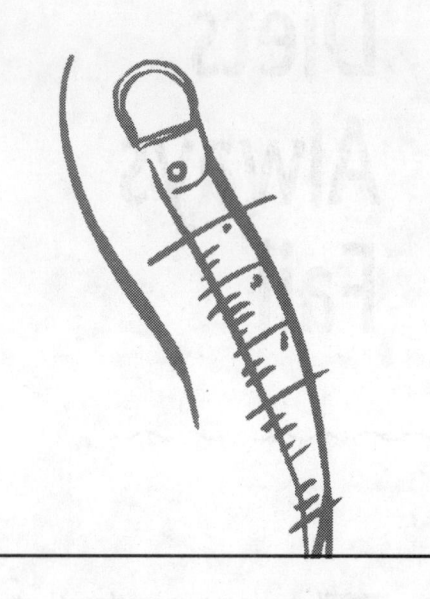

Myth No. 4 ● *It's Hereditary and There's Nothing I Can Do About It*

It's true that heredity is a factor in obesity and even in the pattern of fatness. But it's also true that environmental factors such as the type of food you eat and the exercise you do are more important.

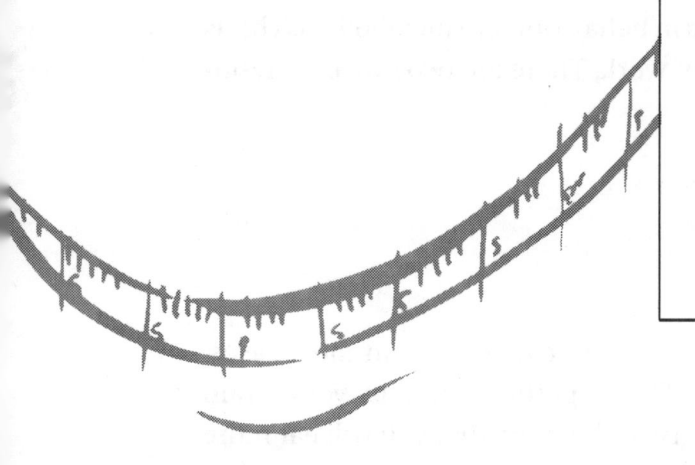

Myth No. 5 ● *Don't Eat Between Meals*

There is strong evidence that you burn up more energy by eating the same number of kilojoules as small meals throughout the day, rather than three square meals.

Why Diets Always Fail

There is no question that dieting doesn't work. If you need evidence of this, I'm sure yourself and friends you know can confirm it. You may lose weight for a short period of time while you're on a diet but, as night follows day, you will not only put the weight back on again, you will actually have more fat than before your diet.

Statistics from the United States tell us that of the people who go on a diet, 95 per cent will regain the weight they lost or put on even more weight within one year and the five per cent who did keep it off were actually worse off for it. They tended to feel depressed, had a hard time tolerating cold, and suffered from constant hunger. In other words, long-term, forced weight loss causes marked alterations in behaviour and metabolism. This is conclusive proof that dieting does not work. There are two proven physiological reasons for this.

WHY DIETING FAILS

1 When you reduce the amount of food you eat you are, in most cases, restricting your nutrient intake. The appetite centre in your brain responds by making you feel hungry in the hope that you will eat more food to satisfy your nutrient requirements. You may resist your hunger feeling for some time but, eventually, your body's instincts will win and you will return to your old eating habits. There is a solution to this which we'll come back to later. The solution works in harmony with your

body's natural physiology and instincts, instead of trying to fight it as dieting does.
2 There is another even more important physiological fact which explains why dieting fails. When you go on a diet you certainly lose weight but only half the weight you lose is fat—the other half is lean muscle. This is the big drawback of dieting—half your weight loss is muscle loss. When you jump on the scales they only give you the good news—the loss of weight. They don't tell you the bad news—the loss of muscle. This loss of lean muscle is disastrous for both your health and your weight problem.

HOW DIETING MAKES YOU FATTER

The loss of muscle due to dieting may mean that you never achieve your goal of becoming slimmer. It will make losing more fat far more difficult and, once you start going back to a more normal diet, you may actually gain more fat than you initially had. You've probably observed this phenomenon yourself. In fact, the five-year follow-up records of every type of diet program show that up to one half of the dieters regained more weight than they lost. During the first year dieters tend to adhere strictly to their diet and therefore the bad effects of dieting are most severe at this time (96 per cent of dieters regain or put on more weight). Over a five-year period people go off and on diets and so the effects are slightly less severe.

Most people who have tried dieting to lose weight have tried several times. The three most common results for dieters are that:
1 They give up the diet since it affects their health or just doesn't work.
2 After the diet they put on more weight than before the diet.
3 Their weight problem gets worse after each new diet—the so-called yo-yo dieting effect.

There are two simple scientific facts which explain why dieting makes you fatter.

First, muscle has a higher metabolic rate than fat, that is, it burns up kilojoules more easily than fat. Now, since dieting causes your body to lose a lot of its muscle the total body metabolic rate has been reduced. This means your body burns up kilojoules slower than before dieting, and the extra kilojoules not burnt up are stored as fat in your body. In fact, the single factor that reduces your metabolic rate more than any other is dieting itself.

Second, the body tends to regard dieting as a form of starvation and will preserve its fat reserves in case the dieting is prolonged. This is a physiological emergency mechanism, whereby the body will sacrifice its protein to provide energy before it will use up its fat reserves. So, you end up with relatively more fat and less protein (muscle) in the body. This explains why dieters often look and feel weak. They also often start to look emaciated and gaunt due to the loss of facial muscles. It's also not uncommon for dieters to start losing their hair, since hair consists mainly of protein.

The body interprets a diet as being a famine and a threat to its survival. Consequently the body automatically and drastically reduces the number of kilojoules it uses for its basic functions. For example, a 74 kilogram person uses around 300 kilojoules an hour while sleeping but this drops dramatically to 170 kilojoules an hour when dieting.

Within two days of beginning a very strict diet the metabolic rate slows by around 15 per cent and fat storage becomes more efficient. Diets simply prepare the body for more efficient storage of fat.

You have a funny kind of problem: your body doesn't realise you are dieting to try to lose fat. The body is only concerned with its number one instinct, which is survival, and it will attempt to preserve its fat supplies for this purpose.

The body actually is remarkably adapted for survival. In the first instance, the body sacrifices its protein supplies for energy before its fat supplies. This is because protein comes from the structure of the body and the body regards its direct energy supply (fat) as being more important in a potential starvation situation. The vital organs—the brain, heart, lungs—all require energy to function, and the body rightly gives this a higher priority than maintaining muscle structure (protein) even though this may cause muscular weakness. The body has another survival mechanism too, in that it uses up its protein supply from the least important structures first. On a restrictive diet, the body will take protein from the hair and muscles first, and only from the vital organs if the diet is prolonged.

There are still more reasons why dieting makes you fatter. These are:
- The loss of muscle tissue from dieting makes you weaker and less active because it is muscle which gives strength to the body. Since you are weaker, you will be less inclined to exercise and this will cause a further build-up of fat.
- Loss of muscle tissue means loss of protein. The enzymes which break down fat to produce energy are made up of protein. Since you have less protein, you will also have fewer enzymes and therefore less fat will be burnt up.
- The body responds to loss of fat by converting some of its protein to fat to correct any imbalance. Some fat is vital for survival and if you lose too much, which is what happens on a strict diet, the body's response is dramatic.

HOW REPEATED DIETING MAKES YOU FATTER STILL

In a survey of 15 000 readers of a major women's magazine, 42 per cent of the overweight readers said they were on again/off again dieters (yo-yo dieters). They lose weight then gain. They are always dieting even when they're gaining and their weight baseline continues to rise.

As far back as 1938, British scientists found that the laboratory rats deprived of food and then allowed to feed freely quickly regained weight and became heavier than rats that had never dieted. They called this rebound 'over-compensation'.

Other early studies found that as weight goes down we lose both fat and protein, but regained weight is largely fat. Cattle raisers have capitalised on this research. By underfeeding animals before fattening them, they have a cheap way of increasing the fat content of beef.

How does yo-yo dieting produce the increased fat? During a diet fat cells shrink; they never disappear. When normal eating is resumed, the fat cells don't just fill up with fat: they multiply, even doubling in number. The new fat cells are very hard to get rid of and they encourage your body to accumulate more fat.

Yo-yo dieting has also been shown to be bad for your health. Jean Mayer, a pioneer in obesity research, put laboratory mice on a feast-fast program and found that yo-yoing shortened their lives. Other researchers put pigs through wide weight swings. The animals developed high blood pressure and heart disease. Another study, done in Massachusetts, involved 5000 men and women over a thirty-year period. One of its findings was that the people whose weight went up and down most had significantly greater chances of dying and, in particular, were especially vulnerable to coronary heart disease.

To sum up, diets don't work. You will inevitably get hungry and miss the old food you used to enjoy. Eventually you will binge to fulfil your cravings. Then you'll feel guilty and diet again. This cycle will continue and before long you will be fatter than you were originally. Your health will suffer and, as you can now plainly see, all the self-discipline and sacrifice will have been for nothing.

To achieve permanent weight loss you need to employ the correct, scientific methods of losing fat, without losing muscle and your health. This book will fulfil that objective.

In the next few chapters, you will be shown how easily fat can be lost on a permanent basis by following the double fat-burning program.

WHERE THE DIET BOOKS HAVE GONE WRONG

Most diet books make two false assumptions.
1. They assume that dieting has no effect on your metabolic rate (i.e. how fast your body burns up its fat).
2. They assume all the weight you lose is fat.

Both of these assumptions are wrong for all the reasons outlined above.

WHAT ACTUALLY HAPPENS WHEN YOU DIET?

Diet books either tell you or imply that when you go on a diet your body starts to burn up its fat reserves in order to provide energy. In reality this does not happen. In the initial stage of a diet, the body draws on the energy that is immediately available. This immediate energy source is glycogen. This is a carbohydrate which is stored in solution with water in the muscles and liver. As glycogen is being used up to provide energy, water from the body's tissues is also being used up. So any initial weight loss is due to the *loss of water*.

If the diet is continued, the body will start to draw on its fat and muscle tissues to produce energy. So from then on a good part of any weight loss is healthy lean muscle. To make matters worse, if you are overweight and don't exercise, you will lose more muscle than a slimmer, more active person. This is because exercise stimulates muscle production, while burning up fat.

WHAT HAPPENS WHEN YOU STOP THE DIET?

When you cease dieting you'll probably start to gain weight straight away. Perhaps you are thinking, 'why not just stay on the diet?' Experience shows that the vast majority of dieters give up their diet. This is understandable, since dieters usually experience a decline in their health, feel tired, depressed and feel they are missing out on their favourite food. A lot of this is due to insufficient nutrients and loss of muscle tissue.

There are a couple of complications when you stop dieting. In the first place, you are so hungry that you tend to overeat and also eat your favourite high-kilojoule foods which you've been missing out on. This tends to become a habit and quite often you end up eating more than before you started dieting. So, of course, you will not only regain any weight you lost, but you will put on more weight. The other problem when you stop dieting is that the extra weight you put on is fat. This is because the dieting has caused your body to reduce its metabolic rate to try to conserve its fat reserves and consequently your body is unable to burn up its fat reserves to produce energy as efficiently as before the diet. This principle will also make future dieting even less successful and reduce the efficiency of your body's ability to burn up fat even more.

After the diet, since your body is less efficient at burning up fat, you will have to eat *less* just to maintain your present weight.

As you can see from the above discussion, ultimately dieting makes you fatter. Fortunately there is a way out of this dilemma. Correct exercise and eating the correct foods will cause you to lose fat without losing muscle. You don't have to diet or even give up all the foods you enjoy. The only way to lose fat will be discussed in the next few chapters.

HOW DIETING CAUSES HEALTH PROBLEMS

Dieting is disastrous to your health for several reasons:
- Since dieting causes muscle loss, you will become weaker and less active because muscle is essential for strength.
- Less muscle tissue also means less protein in your body. Protein is essential for the structure and repair of body tissues and for the physiological and biochemical processes which occur in the body. Enzymes, which are so essential for all the chemical activity in the body including the breakdown of fat to produce energy, are made of protein.
- If you are following a very strict diet you run the risk of not getting sufficient vitamins and minerals. The fact is that you need a sufficient amount of food to obtain sufficient vitamins and minerals.
- On a diet the increased burning of fat causes increased free radical activity, which results in tissue damage and accelerated ageing. With exercise, the fat is replaced by healthy lean muscle which prevents free radical activity.

Free radicals are highly unstable, highly reactive molecules or fragments of molecules with an unpaired free electron which tries to combine with other molecules. Free radicals are usually toxic oxygen molecules that severely damage most of the molecules they combine with. They are produced as the by-product of metabolic processes, or enter the body in food or polluted air.

These free radicals are very destructive; they damage our cells, interfere with DNA replication and can cause cancer. Hence the importance of avoiding severe diets to prevent the burning up of fat too rapidly. Repeated dieting will make matters much worse by repeatedly releasing free radicals.

The body tries to protect itself from these free radicals with free radical scavengers. Some of these scavengers are obtained in food, for example vitamin C, and the element selenium. These scavengers are called anti-oxidants. Reducing your food intake means that you have less protection against free radical damage.

- Another danger of dieting is malnutrition, since dieters often give up foods with high natural fat content, such as nuts, avocadoes and eggs. These foods are very nutritious, being a rich source of vitamins and minerals.

Let's look at eggs as an example. While they do have a high saturated fat content, they also contain a substance called lecithin, which breaks down fat. Eggs are also loaded with nutrients. They are rich in protein, vitamins and minerals. They contain the amino acid, cysteine, which helps prevent premature ageing, including wrinkles, by reducing the cross-linking of collagen fibres that is responsible for ageing the skin. Eggs have a high vitamin B content and, in combination with cysteine, have been shown to increase sexual virility. The lecithin in eggs reduces your cholesterol and feeds your brain, nervous system and glands. Lecithin is one of the most essential nutrients for nerve tissue and the brain comprises very concentrated nerve tissue. A survey of people in their eighties who displayed a high level of mental ability and an active sex life showed that they all consumed eggs on a daily basis. If you don't eat enough eggs every week, you are probably not getting sufficient lecithin in your diet. This leads to an insufficient breakdown of saturated fat from animal foods, such as meat, butter and cheese. The end result is a build-up of fat and cholesterol in your arteries. The advice you hear about giving up eggs if you have a high cholesterol level is obviously incorrect. I would recommend eating about six eggs a week—preferably boiled rather than fried.

In summary, dieting does not work. In the next few chapters you will be shown what does work. You will see how by doing the right type of exercise your body will increase its metabolic rate, not only during the exercise period but for the whole day, even while you are sleeping. The exercise program in this book is designed to have a double fat-burning effect. You will also be shown how the correct nutritional program, based on scientific principles, is essential to achieve fat loss.

The Mental Aspect of Slimming

Everything we do in life has a mental aspect. This applies especially to an area like slimming where motivation and self-discipline are involved. Knowing how to lose fat is only half the battle. The other half is the mental aspect, that is, really wanting to lose weight and being prepared to exercise some discipline in achieving this goal.

Being overweight will probably make you feel unhappy about yourself. This should be the motivation to make you want to lose weight. Once you start to lose weight, you will realise this program works, feel happier and be motivated to keep the program up.

Below you will find the best mental techniques for losing fat.

THE RIGHT ATTITUDE

When you make up your mind to lose weight you will probably approach it in one of two ways. You can either hate the idea of being fat or love the idea of being healthy. The latter attitude is the more positive.

Hating the idea of being fat is what makes chronic dieters continuously starve themselves. If you love the idea of being healthy, you wouldn't do this because you'd realise you would compromise your health. You would also switch your diet from a high fat/sugar diet to a high complex carbohydrate one, since this is the healthy way to lose weight.

By hating the idea of being fat, we place fatness in the centre stage of our mind, which creates fear and negative thinking. By loving the idea of being healthy, we place the image of health at centre stage. This creates a pleasant, positive image to aim for.

The best attitude to adopt is to try and maintain a healthy diet, that is, one high in complex carbohydrates—you will increase your health level and, as a welcome extra bonus, become slimmer.

STUDY YOURSELF

Why is it that you feel satisfied by eating healthy foods like fruit and vegetables one day and the next day binge on junk food? Food may be a solace, a response to boredom, or eating may be just something you do in your spare time. You can only begin to make changes by understanding the emotions and situations that lead you to overeat.

Many people find the evening a tempting time for overeating. This is usually due to a combination of being bored and having food readily available in the kitchen. To help combat this, as soon as you find the television boring, turn it off and do something else. Take a walk or read a book—anything to take your mind off food.

Think about when you are most likely to overeat. Is it at a certain time of day? In a certain place? Is it on weekends or special occasions? By knowing where your weakness is you can develop a technique to overcome it.

CHANGING HABITS

Big advances in behavioural management of weight control over the last decade have seen a number of changes introduced into weight control programs as standard practice. These are as follows:

Stimulus Control

Your aim is to modify any stimulus which has become an automatic cue associated with eating behaviour. This applies to three situations.

Social Situations
- Don't drink alcohol while eating—have it before or after.
- Drink a glass of water, cup of tea etc., instead of having a second serve of the main dish.
- Go to low-fat restaurants (e.g. Japanese, Thai).
- Park away from a restaurant and walk.
- Focus on your behaviour rather than on your weight.
- Plan high-risk situations in advance.

- At a buffet, allow yourself only one trip to the food and use only a small plate.

At Home
- Don't keep high-fat snack foods, chocolate etc., in the fridge.
- Store food out of sight.
- Confine eating to one place in the house (e.g. dining table).
- Leave the table after eating.
- Don't associate anything else with eating (e.g. reading, TV).
- Wait for five minutes in the middle of a meal before eating anything more.
- Eat meals off a smaller plate.
- Always try to leave something on your plate.

Drinking Alcohol
- Don't start drinking until a set time of day (e.g. 7.00 p.m.).
- Have at least one or two 'alcohol-free days'.
- Don't have peanuts or chips in the house.
- Don't drink while eating.
- Combine water/mineral water chasers with alcohol.

Response Management

Your aim is to modify your automatic response to a situation, for example eating at a particular time even if you're not hungry.
- Check your habits.
- Substitute an alternative for eating (walk, drink water, relaxation/meditation).

Reinforcement

Give yourself a reward to reinforce your achievements and encourage yourself to keep going. Read 'Positive Reinforcement Techniques' on page 31.

Self-monitoring

This has probably been the single most valuable finding in behavioural techniques. It involves recording such things as food intake, exercise, eating behaviour, times and moods etc. For example:
- Place a sign on the fridge 'Think before eating'.
- Measure waist size regularly (i.e. weekly).
- Keep an eating diary and identify triggers for eating.

You will become very conscious of your old bad habits—seeing them clearly makes it easier to change them. Bad habits have to be brought from the unconscious to the conscious level of awareness.

LEARN HOW TO RELEASE STRESS

Stress causes weight gain in two ways. In the first instance, **eating triggers the release of endorphins from the brain, which results in a feeling of pleasure.** This is normal. The problem occurs when stress or an emotional problem causes irregularities in the release of the endorphins resulting in an excessive pleasure drive, hence an addiction to sugar. Secondly, **stress makes you want relief, so you eat sweet food to feel better.** This only complicates the situation, since after the initial stimulation, **sugar causes you to feel down.**

One of the best ways to combat this problem, is to learn to **get pleasure from other things, such as having goals, socialising, projects and hobbies.**

It's also important that you don't turn to quick fixes to relieve stress. These often produce short-term, temporary relief but usually increase your stress level in the long run. The quick fixes commonly used are: **coffee; cigarettes; alcohol; tranquillisers; and sleeping pills.**

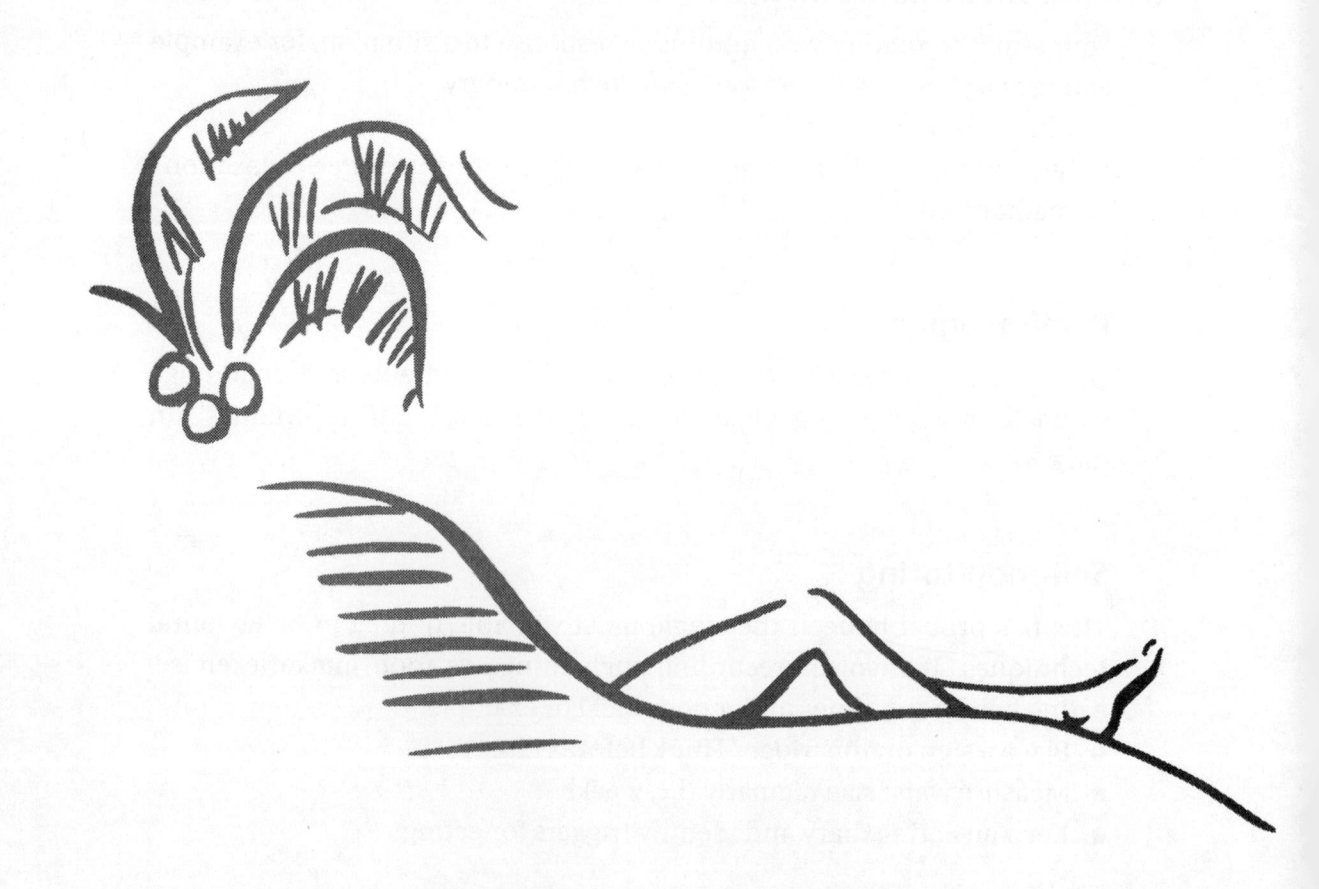

Ten Ways to Handle Stress

1 ● Positive Attitude

People often attribute stress and the discomfort they experience to some external factor. In reality, studies have shown that stress is mainly an internal factor—it's how we personally react to a situation which causes the discomfort, and not the external situation itself.

One person may react to a situation by considering it to be a problem and worrying about it. Another person considers the same situation as a challenge and looks forward to meeting it face on. The external situation is the same and yet one person experiences stress and the other person doesn't. Obviously stress is an internal factor and depends on your attitude rather than the event itself.

The solution is to think positively about any situation, since most potential 'disasters' don't happen anyway. You are better off taking positive steps to prevent or remedy a problem rather than worry about it.

2 ● Live a More Relaxed Life

It is important to slow down—stop rushing around—you will achieve just as much, if not more. In short, take it easy.

3 ● Exercise

Aerobic exercise releases stress and induces a feeling of relaxation. Many studies have shown that exercise does reduce anxiety levels and depression. One recent American study compared the effect of stress on two groups of students. One group had completed a 14-week aerobic program; the other had not. Each group was asked to solve a set of mostly insolvable problems. The exercise group displayed a much lower level of muscle tension and anxiety than the non-exercise group.

4 ● Laughing

Laughing has long been known to release stress, as well as being enjoyable. Research verifies this fact. Laughing increases respiratory exchange and heart-rate. It also stimulates the production of beta-endomorphines which are the same chemicals that produce the runner's 'high'. In fact, laughing can be regarded as 'internal jogging'.

There are several well documented cases of people making a total recovery from terminal cancer just by watching hilarious videos. Laughter is certainly the best medicine, and it's free. Laughing requires no training or equipment—you just need to cultivate a sense of humour.

5 ● *Crying*

Studies show that crying reduces stress. In one study, a group of people with stress-related disorders were compared with a group of healthy people of similar age and background. One major difference found was that the healthy group was not ashamed to cry, whereas the sick group regarded crying as a sign of weakness or loss of control. In one survey, 73 per cent of the men and 85 per cent of the women questioned stated they felt better after crying.

6 ● *Set Realistic Goals*

One of the most common causes of stress occurs when people cannot see that the goals that they have set themselves are beyond them, and they need to readjust their sights. The so-called 'mid-life crisis', when stress disorders reach epidemic proportions, is usually due to setting unrealistic goals.

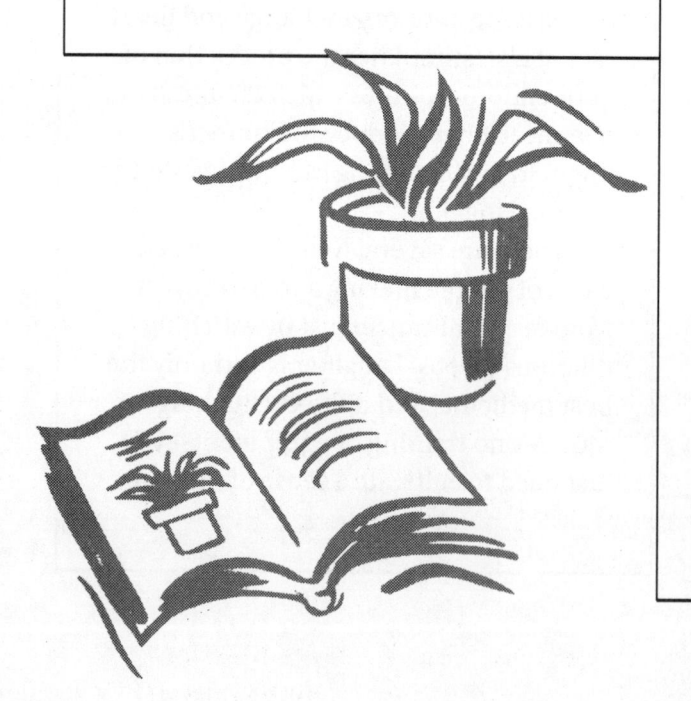

7 ● *Recreation*

This is a very apt word since it literally means to re-create, that is, to change activity and become more creative. If you spend too long on any one activity, even if you enjoy the activity, you are likely to feel stressed. Vary your activities and spend more time doing such things as sport, gardening, reading, hobbies and socialising.

If you need to spend a long time on one particular activity, take small breaks and do something else.

Don't view recreation as a waste of time. If you work too hard with not enough recreation, you will become stressed and you may turn to food as a quick fix.

8 ● *Increase Your Vitality Level*

Your vitality level is one of the most effective factors in coping with stress. If your vitality level is high, you can handle stress and you'll tend to view events more as a challenge, rather than stress. If you're feeling good, life takes on a different perspective. If stressful situations do arise, you have the energy and clarity of mind to overcome them. You can't always avoid stress, but you can increase your vitality level so that you can cope with stress.

To increase your vitality level, follow the nutritional and exercise guidelines in this book. If you're really interested in this topic, you can also read another book I've written called *Reversing Ageing*.

9 ● Social Relationships

Many studies have shown that separations from other family members, especially by death or divorce, are the most stressful events in life. Fortunately it also works the other way; support from people around you can have an equally powerful effect in reducing stress.

Studies have shown that social support causes an increase in lifespan, reduces stress following the loss of a loved one, speeds recovery from surgery and heart attack, and alleviates the symptoms of asthma and other disorders.

10 ● Relaxation Techniques

Studies show that people who set a little time aside each day to do a relaxation technique or meditate have lower stress levels.

For details of these techniques, again read *Reversing Ageing* (see 'Further Reading').

POSITIVE REINFORCEMENT TECHNIQUES

These techniques are designed to help you use rewards to increase your weight loss motivation and drive.

Research shows that any behaviour followed by a reward is more likely to be repeated. This means that the more you are rewarded (by yourself and others) for your weight loss efforts, the more likely you are to succeed and the easier the task will be.

Reward Yourself

Reward yourself daily for your achievement in reducing high fat/sugar foods. Replace the pleasures of eating your favourite dish with more simple pleasures—a walk in the park, reading a good book or ringing up a good friend.

Use the money you save on high fat/sugar dishes and fast foods to treat yourself. Every week, buy yourself some items of clothing, go to the cinema or buy a large quantity of your favourite fruit.

Not only will you enjoy these rewards but you know you deserve them, and it will give you incentive to keep up the slimming program.

Positive Self-talk

By talking positively to yourself, you'll increase your determination and resolve to be in control of your eating behaviour. When you find yourself wanting to eat at an inappropriate time or experience excessive cravings, silently repeat one or two positive messages to yourself several times. For example you can assert, 'I will not eat this fattening food' and 'I am in control'.

These messages are called positive affirmations, and are very effective in achieving goals.

Mirror Talk

Have a heart-to-heart talk with yourself while standing in front of a mirror. Repeat your positive affirmations while looking in the mirror.

Creative Imagination

Just before you fall asleep, imagine yourself eating small portions of food and chewing the food very slowly. See yourself in control and saying no to high fat/sugar foods which were once your weakness. Picture yourself eating low fat/sugar nutritious foods, such as fruit salad and vegetables.

Also imagine the rewards of your eating discipline—looking slimmer, wearing smaller sized clothes, getting compliments, having more energy and feeling good about yourself.

This technique is very effective, since it plants new images in your brain which will affect your actions quite automatically. What you are really doing is using auto-suggestion to communicate with your subconscious mind. The ideal time to communicate with your subconscious is just before sleep when you are feeling slightly drowsy (your conscious mind is turning off). At this time there is no interference from the conscious mind. You are actually in a natural hypnotic trance state. Any suggestion made at this time—verbal or visual—will go straight through to your subconscious mind.

It's best to do this exercise as soon as you get into bed, since if you wait too long you will probably fall asleep before starting the exercise.

Improvement Diary

Keep a record of the improvements you experience in your mental and physical health as you begin to lose fat. You'll notice you have more energy, sleep better and look younger. Your old tight clothes will start to fit you again.

You'll also experience mental improvements. You will feel more confident, have a better self-image and experience a sense of achievement, pride and self-control.

In addition you can utilise the self-discipline you have developed to improve in other areas of your life—such as stopping smoking.

EXERCISE IMPROVES YOUR MENTAL STATE

Exercise increases the blood supply to your whole body including your brain and face. This means you feel good and look good. In addition, when you look good you feel better about yourself.

When you feel good, you are more inclined to eat right. It's when you are low that you start reaching for high sugar snacks to give you a lift.

HOW TO HANDLE RELAPSES

Making the change to a new healthier and slimmer lifestyle is not difficult. The greatest challenge is keeping it up.

Don't worry if you have the occasional relapse—everybody does. Just see these relapses as isolated slip-ups, not as total catastrophes. Instead of viewing your diet relapses as defeats, try to learn from them. Note the sequence of events that preceded them.

Most relapses occur when you are under stress, so adopt the points above for preventing stress.

Successful Slimming for Females

Weight gain in females over 35 is partly due to a slowing down of the metabolic rate and partly due to the decline in exercise that comes with age. Beginning in their 30s, many women find themselves very busy yet less physically active than ever before.

PREGNANCY

By the mid 30s many women are having their last children and increasing numbers are having their first. According to Robin Kanarek, a physiological psychologist at Tufts University, Medford, Massachusetts 'Some women feel that during pregnancy, they finally have permission to eat whatever they want'. Of course this means they gain weight.

There is also the common phenomenon of gaining an extra two or three kilograms after a pregnancy. This extra two to three kilograms is extremely difficult to lose. Weight loss is even more difficult if you have had several pregnancies, due to the 'yoyo' phenomenon. Yoyo-ing means that you gain and lose weight several times over a period of years, as occurs with pregnancies. Whenever you gain weight, more comes back as fat and less as lean muscle. Since fat has a lower metabolic rate than muscle, the whole body's metabolic rate is lowered, resulting in less fat being burnt up.

THE EMPTY NEST SYNDROME

Older women often face the stress of loneliness when children leave home or because of divorce or widowhood. Loneliness and boredom tend to make people overeat.

As a replacement for the pleasure of company, women may turn to the pleasure derived from eating foods high in sugars and fats such as cakes and sweets. Sugar also gives you a short, temporary lift helping to alleviate boredom and depression. My best advice is to follow the exercise program in this book because the mental lift it gives you will be more pleasant and sustained. The exercise program also gives you a feeling of doing something constructive to improve yourself, and adds some structure to the day.

MENOPAUSE

Menopause is another time when a weight gain may occur. Studies show that menopause itself does not cause weight gain. However, menopause does cause an unhealthy shift in the places where fat is stored and this, combined with a reduction in physical activity at around this age, can lead to excessive weight gain. Yale biochemist Marielle Rebuffe-Scrive has found that the activity of a certain kind of enzyme called lipoprotein-lipase—which helps attract fat to wherever it resides—declines in the hips and thighs after menopause. Meanwhile another enzymatic process called lipolysis—which makes it easy to get rid of fat—is reduced in the upper body of post-menopause women. These enzyme changes are the result of reduced levels of the female hormones, oestrogen and progesterone. The overall effect of these changes in enzyme activity is to increase fat in the upper part of the body.

THE SOLUTION

For all women regardless of their age, the same principles for losing fat apply. You need to do correct exercise and replace some of your fats and sugars with complex carbohydrate food (fruits, vegetables and wholegrains), as explained in other chapters of the book.

Seek out pleasures and activities unrelated to food if you tend to overeat. A lot of people who think they want food really want pleasure, solace, comfort and relief from boredom. For people in this category, remember that food is only one of many different types of pleasures. Instead of taking a food 'fix', try the pleasure of taking a hot bath, taking a long peaceful walk, reading a good book, calling a friend, socialising, planning a holiday and so on.

If you still find you are having problems in this area, don't hesitate to get counselling. Sometimes we are too close to ourselves to see a solution. A third party can often help us understand ourselves better.

Common Questions About Weight Control

✱ *How Quickly Can I Lose Weight?*

You may be wondering how quickly you will lose weight. This depends entirely on how quickly you want to lose weight.

If you wish to lose weight quickly (about one kilogram per week) you will need to give up all high fat/sugar foods for a while and you will need to exercise six times a week. If you are over thirty years of age, you should do different types of exercise on alternate days. For example do the double fat-burning exercises on Mondays, Wednesdays and Fridays, and some form of aerobic exercise (walking, jogging, aerobics) on Tuesdays, Thursdays and Saturdays. This prevents straining the same muscles.

If you wish to be more moderate in your lifestyle (you may want to exercise only four times a week and not give up all your favourite foods), you will lose about one kilogram per month.

Both the fast way and the slower way are safe, since you will be eating nutritious food and merely giving up or reducing excess fat and sugar. This is not dieting. Even exercising six days a week will not place any strain on your body, as long as you do different exercises on alternate days.

I don't recommend trying to lose more than one kilogram per week. To do more than this you will have to go on an extreme crash diet where you will be losing lean muscle and water as well as fat. This is what most of the current diets do and it is harmful to health. Furthermore, you will eventually become even fatter (see 'How Dieting Makes You Fatter', page 19).

Don't be surprised if you reach a stage where you don't seem to be losing any more weight. If you are faithfully keeping the program up, this is a good sign. It means your body is replacing the excess fat with lean muscle. You are still losing fat, it's just turning to healthy lean muscle. Since muscle has a higher metabolic rate than fat, your body will now start to burn up even more fat.

So, you can see that weighing yourself is not really an accurate indication of fat loss. The harmful crash diets will show you are losing weight but most of this weight loss is healthy muscle and water, not fat.

A far more accurate method of assessing fat loss is to measure your waistline. This is where you have 100 per cent excess fat. Any loss here is purely fat. I suggest, instead of aiming to lose one kilogram a week or month, you aim to lose 2.5 centimetres (1 inch) a week or month from your waistline.

✳ Why Do Women Get Fat Bottoms and Men Get Fat Tummies?

Women have more fat cells around their bottoms and thighs, whereas men's fat cells are distributed more evenly. In addition, there is a chemical in the body which accelerates the flow of fat cells. In women, more of this chemical is in the bottom and thighs, so they tend to store fat there. Men store fat around their internal abdominal organs.

✳ Why Can Some People Eat a Lot and Still Not Get Fat?

Different metabolic rates, genetic factors and activity patterns all combine to give us different energy requirements. If you follow the program in this book, you will be able to eat a lot and still lose fat. This is because your metabolic rate will be higher and you will be eating more nourishing food.

✳ Does Obesity Affect My Health?

Most definitely. You have far more chance of developing the following conditions: high blood pressure; kidney disease; coronary heart problems; cerebral haemorrhage; diabetes; arthritis; gallstones; gout; many cancers; haemorrhoids; back trouble; and psychological problems.

Your chances of surgery are also increased. Fat people undergo operations two to four times as often as those of normal weight.

✹ *Is It A Good Idea To Eat Before Bedtime?*

It's best to avoid eating before bedtime. You will be sleeping for the next eight hours or so which means that the fat and sugar from the food cannot be used up as energy: it will be stored as fat instead.

✹ *Is It Safe To Take Weight Loss Preparations?*

In general it's best to stay away from artificial preparations. Most don't work; some do but they work by interfering with the body's normal physiology.

The only safe and sure way to lose fat is by replacing high fat/sugar foods with low fat/sugar nutritious foods, and doing the double fat-burning exercises and aerobic exercises.

✹ *Aren't Fat People Supposed To Be Happy People?*

This is a common myth. How could you be happy if you look unattractive and have much more chance of getting one or more of the health problems listed above.

In addition, being just slightly overweight (say, three kilograms) is equivalent to carrying around a 3 kilogram weight attached to your belt all day. Imagine how tired that would make you feel and how it would slow you down. In effect, that's what you are doing when you are overweight. Imagine the extra work on your heart, all day and every day of the year.

✹ *How Can I Control My Appetite?*

There are three main ways to do this.
1. Eat nutritious low fat/sugar food. This will satisfy your body's needs for nutrients quickly and consequently satisfy your appetite much more quickly than if you ate processed or junk food.
2. Eat snacks throughout the day. If you don't do this, your blood sugar level will go down and you will feel very hungry and crave sweet things. If you have cravings, you will tend to overeat and eat high kilojoule sugar foods. Eat healthy snacks, such as fruit.
3. Eat slowly. This increases the nourishment to your body and thus reduces your appetite.

Part Two

The Double Fat-Burning Exercise Program

How the Double Fat-Burning Exercise Program Works

CORRECT EXERCISE—THE ONLY SCIENTIFIC AND HEALTHY WAY TO BECOME SLIM

Correct exercise is the secret to eliminating fat because it increases your metabolic rate which in turn increases your fat-burning capacity. Not only does correct exercise do this while you are exercising but it actually increases your metabolic rate all day, even while you are sleeping.

Two Types of Exercise Which Burn Fat

There are two types of exercise which increase your metabolic rate and fat-burning capacity.

Aerobic exercise Aerobic exercises are fitness-type exercises such as jogging, brisk walking, aerobics, cycling, swimming. It is essential to do this type of exercise properly to achieve optimum results. You will be shown this in the next chapter.

Muscle-stimulating (strength) exercise Muscle-stimulating exercises are body-building exercises such as lifting weights, isometric and isotonic exercises.

Women needn't be put off doing this type of exercise since it includes gentle exercises such as chair-stepping, rowing machines and even stomach sit-up exercises come under this category. You won't develop bulky muscles because you are emphasising low-effort repetition of exercises rather than power exercises. Also, the female hormone system is not geared to produce big, bulky muscles; instead you will develop a lean firm, more contoured body.

In men, muscle-stimulating exercises will produce bulkier, stronger muscles since this type of exercise stimulates the male hormone testosterone. You can control the extent of body building you desire, by emphasising power or repetition. This increase in testosterone further stimulates muscle growth giving you an even greater fat-burning capacity. Incidentally, increased testosterone will also increase the sex drive of both males and females, since females also have small amounts of testosterone.

In essence, if you are a male you will look more masculine and if you are female you will look more feminine.

WHY THE DOUBLE FAT-BURNING PROGRAM IS ESSENTIAL FOR FAT LOSS

Studies show that people who do 'lower body exercise' (mostly walkers and runners) lose upper body strength and muscle mass as they age. This means as you age you are developing a higher fat to muscle ratio. In other words, your body has a higher proportion of fat and since fat has a lower metabolic rate than muscle, you are burning up less fat as each year goes by. Since the double fat-burning exercise program includes upper body exercises, the fat in this area will be replaced by lean muscle.

The double fat-burning exercises have been carefully selected to exercise the upper and lower body including the abdomen. In fact, most of the exercises work on several parts of the body at the same time making them very time economical. For example, skipping and rowing exercises the arms, chest and legs.

In addition, the double fat-burning exercises stimulate muscle production as well as being aerobic. It is the combination of these two factors that makes the double fat-burning exercises superior to purely aerobic exercises.

HOW THE EXERCISE PROGRAM WORKS

The scientific principle behind slimming is the physiological fact that muscle has a higher metabolic rate than fat. Both aerobic exercises and muscle-stimulating exercises convert fat to muscle. One of your aims on this program is to build more muscle. This increased proportion of muscle to fat means a higher total body metabolic rate.

The Supreme Fat-Burning Exercise Program

Since both aerobic exercises and muscle-stimulating exercises burn up fat, why not do exercises which are both aerobic and muscle-stimulating at the same time and *save* time. This is the exercise program I have developed for this book. It means you have the advantage of the double fat-burning effect for no extra time outlay and attain a firm, toned body as a fringe benefit. It's extremely time economical and produces many benefits.

PROOF THAT EXERCISE MAKES YOU LOSE FAT

Several studies have shown that fatter people do not eat more on average than thinner people. In fact, some investigations, such as a 1979 study of 3454 officeworkers, reveal that fat people eat *less* than slimmer people.

However, studies also show that slim people are more active than fat people. A survey by the Stanford University School of Medicine found that among slim, tennis-playing women (ages 32 to 45 years) playing eleven hour per week, average daily kilojoule intake was 10 116, while among sedentary, moderately overweight women of the same age it was 6236 kilojoules. Here were slim women remaining slim on 62 per cent more kilojoules than overweight women.

In 1973, Dr Grant Gwinup of the University of California decided to experiment with a group of thirty-four overweight patients all demoralised after years of futile attempts to reduce their weight by dieting. He told them not to diet; instead he asked them to walk every day, gradually increasing time and distance.

At first, nothing happened. Then, as their walks edged up past half an hour a day, the patients began to notice a weight loss. By the end of one year, every one of the eleven patients who stayed with the program had lost substantial weight and kept it off. The least successful had shed 4.5 kilograms; the most successful, 17 kilograms; and the average was 10 kilograms.

In another study, forty-eight sedentary men (ages 30 to 35) started on a one-year jogging program. The results of the study were as follows:
- The more the men ran, the greater the loss of body fat.
- The more they ran, the greater their increase in food intake.

In fact, those who ran the most ate the most, yet lost the greatest amount of body fat.

As you can see from these results, exercise works where dieting fails. The basic reason for this is that dieting slows the body's metabolism, while exercise speeds it up.

PROOF OF THE EFFECTIVENESS OF THE DOUBLE FAT-BURNING EXERCISE PROGRAM

Dr James Rippe, a cardiologist and expert in physiology and nutrition, studied changes in body fat and muscle content of sixty-five dieters, split into four groups. On average:

- Non-exercisers lost 4 kilograms but 11 per cent of it was muscle.
- Aerobic exercisers lost 4.5 kilograms and only 1 per cent was muscle.
- Muscle-stimulating exercisers lost 4 kilograms and added 9 per cent to their muscle mass.
- Exercisers who did both aerobic and muscle-stimulating exercises lost nearly 6 kilograms and added 4 per cent to their muscle mass.

Let's look at what's happening here, since this study sums up the whole basis of why the double fat-burning exercise program is the most potent method of slimming that exists. First, the group that dieted with no exercise program actually ended up being worse off because the 11 per cent loss of lean muscle tissue lowered their total body metabolic rate, ultimately resulting in less fat burning. The 4-kilogram loss was only a temporary loss. The aerobic exercisers did well but not as well as the muscle-stimulating exercisers who actually added 9 per cent extra muscle. This extra muscle with its high metabolic rate will burn up more of the body's fat. The group which did both types of exercise lost the most weight (6 kilograms) and all of the loss was fat. The gain of only 4 per cent muscle is actually misleading because this last group did an excessive amount of exercise (both types separately every day) which would have caused some muscle (protein) loss. The double fat-burning exercise program avoids this by doing both types of exercise at the same time, and therefore in half the time of the study group. There is no major assault on the body's muscular system.

THE IMPORTANCE OF MUSCLE FOR LOSING FAT

There are three very important characteristics of muscle which make it ideal for burning up excess fat.

First, muscle burns up a lot of kilojoules because body movement uses more kilojoules than any other body function. Second, a large proportion of the body is composed of muscle, so there is great scope for kilojoule burning. Just these two factors are responsible for muscle burning up 90 per cent of the total kilojoules burnt, even when resting. Third, when we exercise, the fat-burning enzyme in muscle can increase kilojoule burning by fifty-fold.

It is important to remember that the only way fat can be lost is through being burnt up in muscle. This makes you realise how important muscle is for getting rid of excess fat.

If you go on a severe diet, you will not be getting sufficient fat in your diet and your body will use up some of its fat supply. The problem is, some of your muscle protein is also converted to fat. Since you now have less muscle, you also have reduced fat-burning capacity, so you are worse off than before.

When you do aerobic exercises, your muscle burns up more fat without the loss of muscle tissue. This means you end up with a greater proportion of muscle to fat which translates into a greater fat-burning capacity. This is obviously the way to go.

To fully appreciate the importance of muscle, just keep in mind your MUSCLES BURN UP MOST OF THE KILOJOULES YOU EAT.

ENZYMES—THE KEY TO FAT LOSS

Enzymes are specific proteins which have the ability to speed up chemical reactions. They can speed up the breakdown of fat to produce energy so, as you can imagine, they play an essential role in getting rid of your fat.

Fatty acids, either from our fat deposits or from a recent meal, are carried by the blood to muscle cells. Inside the cells, the fat enzymes break up the fatty acids and energy is thereby released.

The enzymes used in fat breakdown need a lot of oxygen. Intense exercise for short periods causes an oxygen deficit, so the fat enzymes cannot operate and fat cannot be broken down. When you exercise at between 75–80 per cent of your maximum pulse rate, your muscles require a lot of oxygen. This allows your fat enzymes to operate and results in the breakdown of fat. Not only this, but aerobic exercise also stimulates the production of more fat enzymes, resulting in even more fat breakdown.

WHAT IS AEROBIC EXERCISE?

This is steady continuous exercise which raises the pulse rate to 75–80 per cent of the maximum pulse rate for your age for at least twenty minutes.

Aerobic exercise has two major effects on the body:
1 It produces a stronger heart and healthier lungs. This results in the cardio-vascular system delivering oxygen more efficiently to every cell in the body (including your fat cells).

2   The muscles become more efficient at absorbing oxygen from the blood, and therefore at converting stored fat to muscle and energy.

AEROBIC EXERCISE AND FAT LOSS

Exercises aimed at specific body parts such as stomach or hip exercises do not cause body fat loss. 'Spot' reducing does not work. Specific body exercises, such as sit-ups, will not cause any fat loss: this has been scientifically proven. Aerobic exercise burns up fat. You will lose fat from all over the body wherever there is excess fat. You will even lose fat from the walls of your arteries. This will improve your health immensely and greatly reduce your risk of suffering from heart disease or having a stroke.

Aerobic Exercise Results In Increased Lean Muscle As Well As Fat Loss

In one research program, eleven overweight university women were put on an eight-week walk-jog program. Even though the women had no dietary restrictions, they lost on average more than two kilograms each. But on the basis of skin-fold measurements and other means the researchers discovered that the women had lost an average of almost 5.5 kilograms of fat each. The difference between the fat loss (5.5 kg) and the actual loss (2 kg) is explained by an increase in lean muscle (more than 2.5 kg). This in itself produced a slimmer look since, being denser, muscle of a given weight takes up less space than an equal weight of fat.

Exercise Also Reduces Sugar Cravings

Exercise stabilises the level of sugar in your blood, lowering it if it is high, or increasing it if it is too low (as is often the case for dieters). When your blood sugar is stable it is easier to reduce high-kilojoule sugar snacks. In addition, because exercise makes you feel better you will be less likely to feel the psychological urge to eat sugar foods.

So next time you feel a craving for more sweet foods, do some exercise: it's far more effective than trying to use your willpower.

Other Benefits of Aerobic Exercise

1 Aerobic exercise makes the heart a more efficient pump, able to meet the demands of strenuous activity with fewer beats because it can pump out more blood with each contraction.

This type of exercise also helps to prevent heart attacks (a reduction of 39 per cent according to one study).

2 The circulation is increased to all parts of the body, resulting in increased efficiency of the internal organs and glands.

3 Blood pressure is reduced.

4 Total blood cholesterol levels are reduced. Perhaps more important, aerobic exercise causes a reduction in the bad low-density cholesterol which clogs the arteries and an increase in the high-density cholesterol which helps to clean the arteries out.

5 Exercise results in fewer health problems and pains.

6 Exercising against gravity (such as walking or running as opposed to swimming) increases the calcium content of bones, helping to prevent osteoporosis and fractures in later life. One study found that women aged sixty-nine to ninety-five years who exercised thirty minutes a day, three days a week for three years, experienced a 2.3 per cent increase in the mineral content of the radius bone in their arms, whereas a group of non-exercisers showed a 3.3 per cent loss.

7 An American study of more than 5000 former university athletes has shown that women who exercise have lower rates of breast and reproductive system cancers.

8 The perspiration from exercise causes increased toxin elimination and healthier skin.

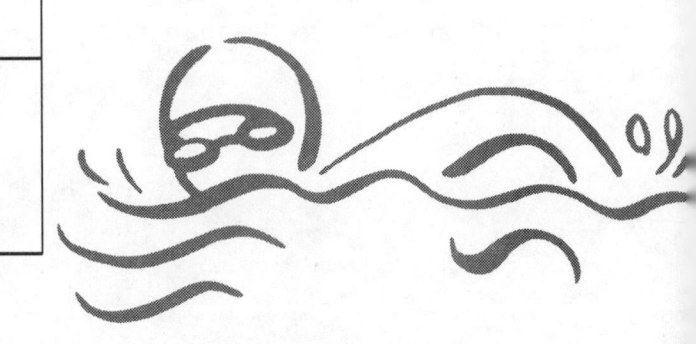

9 Exercise causes a slowing down of the ageing process. One study found that for every one hour of exercise, you'll add two and a half hours to your life. This makes exercise a very good time investment.

10 The nervous system is improved by exercise. According to studies at the University of Texas, sixty-year-old men who have jogged or played squash for twenty years or longer have reaction times equal to, or better than inactive men in their twenties.

11 Exercise is a natural tranquilliser and antidepressant. It releases stress.

Exercise also results in an increase in confidence, optimism and creativity. In a 1985 survey of 1033 men and women, respondents who exercised regularly described themselves as more confident and creative than did their sedentary counterparts.

WHY YOU MUST EXERCISE AS YOU GET OLDER

As you get older, your muscle gradually turns to fat if you don't exercise. Since fat has a lower metabolic rate than muscle, you will burn up fewer kilojoules than when you were younger. This means you will gain even more fat. If you do aerobic exercise, you will gain muscle and this will burn up kilojoules faster (even while you sleep) resulting in loss of fat. It's that simple.

At Stanford University Medical School, researchers tested forty-five healthy men who exercised regularly; most of them were runners. The average percentage of fat contained in their bodies (13 per cent) was the same as for men twenty-five years younger. These results indicate that these active men did not follow the usual process of putting on weight as they grew older.

Why Women Must Put In More Effort

Unfortunately women have to work harder at keeping fat off. In fact, men lose weight faster than women because their muscle-to-fat ratio is naturally higher, and consequently their metabolism is faster. This means exercise is even more important to women than it is to men.

YOU CAN EAT MORE ON THE DOUBLE FAT-BURNING EXERCISE PROGRAM

This exercise program will result in a rapid replacement of fat with muscle, causing you to burn thousands of extra kilojoules per week. This occurs because muscle tissue is more metabolically active than fat tissue. A 70-kilogram person whose weight is mostly lean muscle can eat 2000 kilojoules more per day than someone of the same weight who has more fat than muscle. And this doesn't count the kilojoules burned by exercise sessions themselves.

Once you're in shape from the double fat-burning exercise program you may eat 25 per cent more than before. By contrast, people who don't exercise lose about 225 grams of muscle each year. The kilojoules that would have been burned by muscle end up being stored as fat. That's why you can't afford to over-indulge in your favourite dishes and why you get middle-age spread.

THE THREE PRINCIPLES OF EXERCISE FOR MAXIMUM FAT LOSS

Principle 1
We must lose no muscle, since muscle has a high metabolic rate and burns up fat very efficiently. There are two things which cause muscle loss. These are dieting and doing the same aerobic exercise every day. The body simply doesn't have sufficient time to repair muscle loss from the strain of exercise.

Principle 2
There are only two things which burn up fat without causing loss of muscle. These are aerobic exercises and muscle-stimulating (strength) exercises.

Principle 3
To achieve maximum fat loss in the minimum time, we need to do an exercise system which is both aerobic and muscle-stimulating at the same time.

The double fat-burning exercise system described in this book complies with the above three principles.

How to Exercise Correctly

If you want to gain maximum benefit from the double fat-burning exercise program, you should follow the guidelines in this chapter as carefully as possible.

Experience has shown that many people do not exercise correctly. They often do the wrong type of exercise and even those who do the right type of exercise often do it incorrectly and therefore don't gain optimum results. The next chapter will show you the most potent exercise system for losing fat: so learn the correct approach from this chapter first.

HOW LONG AND HOW OFTEN SHOULD WE EXERCISE—LATEST RESEARCH

Until recently, there has been much controversy about the duration and frequency of exercise. There have been two schools of thought on this. One school says that you need to exercise for at least thirty minutes, three or four days a week. The basis for this thought is that the body doesn't start to burn fat until about twenty minutes into exercise so, logically, you would need to exercise for at least thirty minutes to burn up any significant amount of fat.

The second school of thought states that you need to exercise every day, or at least six days a week, but only for about fifteen minutes. The basis of this thought is that an aerobic exercise session causes an increase in body metabolism for only twenty-four hours after the exercise. This means you have to exercise every day to maintain an increased metabolic rate all day in order to burn up fat all day, every day.

Which school of thought is correct? Actually, both are correct but the second concept is far more effective. It's true that the body doesn't start to burn fat until about twenty minutes after exercising but the amount of fat burnt in the next ten minutes or so of exercise is negligible. If you drink a glass of milk after an exercise session, you immediately replace the fat you lost while exercising. Whenever you exercise, the critical factor is an increased metabolic rate which increases fat burning twenty-four hours a day, every day. Exercising every day for at least fifteen minutes achieves this. Strictly speaking, it takes just twelve minutes of exercise to produce the twenty-four hour effect: but you need to reach your target heart rate first which takes at least three minutes when doing exercises such as jogging and aerobics. Less strenuous exercises such as walking, cycling (outdoor and stationary) and swimming must be done for about eight minutes before the body reaches its target heart rate, so you'll need to exercise for at least twenty minutes (eight minutes plus twelve minutes).

For optimum results, I recommend that you do the double fat-burning exercises for about twenty minutes each session. (See also page 55.)

THE BEST TIME TO EXERCISE

There is no hard and fast rule here; it depends on what's convenient for you. Some like to do it early in the morning when the air is fresh; they claim it gives them energy for the whole day. However, research has shown that early evening is the best time to exercise. This is for three reasons:

1 The whole day's *stress is released*, which induces a feeling of relaxation and vitality.
2 Sleep is improved, due to the release of stress, and that benefits the whole of the next day.
3 Studies have shown that the greatest fat loss and greatest muscle gain can occur with evening exercise. This is probably because appetite is reduced for about two hours after exercise. Eating less in the evening is especially beneficial, since body metabolism is lower in the evening, so you won't burn up the evening meal kilojoules as easily as the other meals.

HOW HARD SHOULD WE EXERCISE?

If you exercise below your target heart rate (see Table 1, page 52), you won't get fit. If you push yourself too hard, you will suffer from fatigue and muscle loss and you won't burn up any fat.

To know exactly how hard to exercise, you just have to take your pulse after exercise. You should aim for a pulse of 80 per cent of your maximum pulse; this will be your target heart rate (T.H.R.). Table 1 (page 52) shows you how to find the 80 per cent level for your age. For example, if you are forty years old, your heart rate (pulse) after exercise should be 146.

You may also use a formula to calculate your target heart rate.

1 Subtract your age from 220.
2 Multiply that figure by 0.8.

If you find after exercise, your pulse is more than six beats below your target heart rate, you'll need to go a little harder. If your pulse is more than six beats above your target heart rate, you'll need to slow down a little.

Don't push yourself too hard, you will lose more than you gain. If you wish to get fit faster, exercise *longer*, not harder.

WHAT IF YOU'RE FIT ALREADY?

If your pulse rate is below sixty at rest, you'll need to revise your target heart rate downwards, since you'll be pushing yourself too hard if you follow the above.

Your revised formula will be:

T.H.R. = (maximum pulse − resting pulse) multiplied by 0.65 + resting pulse

Let's say you are forty years old and your resting pulse rate is 55. The maximum pulse rate for a forty-year old is 182 (from Table 1, page 52). Applying the formula:

$$\text{T.H.R.} = (182 - 55) \times 0.65 + 55 = 137.5$$

DON'T DO THE SAME EXERCISE EVERY DAY IF OVER THIRTY YEARS OLD

If you are over thirty years of age, I recommend that you do the double fat-burning exercises only three days a week, every second day. On the three alternate days, do an aerobic exercise such as walking, jogging or aerobics.

If you do the same exercise every day, you are putting stress on the same muscles every day. Your body doesn't have enough time in between exercise periods to repair the stress. Your muscles will lose structure and become weaker and, as you now know, this is counterproductive! You need those muscles to burn up fat. You may also develop a haggard appearance, as the body draws protein from the face to try to repair the muscles overexercised.

Table 1: Your Target Heart Rate

Age	80% of max. pulse (Target Heart Rate)	75% of max. pulse (heart disease history)	Maximum pulse
20	160	150	200
22	158	148	195
24	157	147	196
26	155	145	194
28	154	144	192
30	152	143	190
32	151	142	189
34	150	140	187
36	149	140	186
38	147	138	184
40	146	137	182
45	143	134	179
50	140	131	175
55	137	128	171
60	128	120	160
65+	120	113	150

Target Heart Rate (if your resting pulse is over 60)

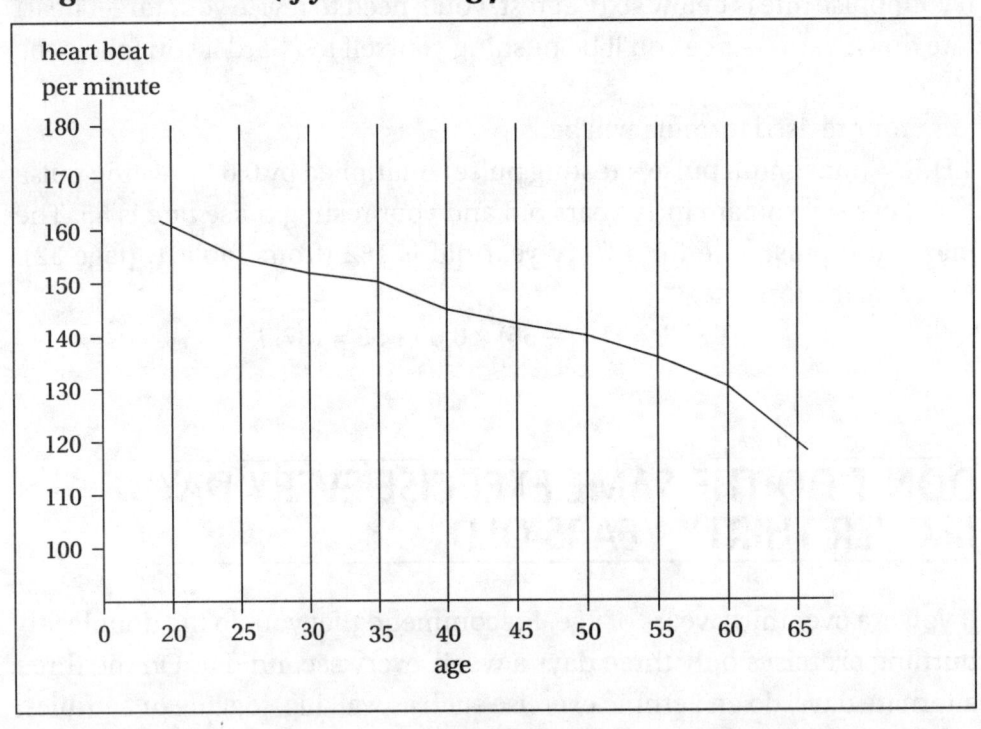

You can use the table or the graph to find your target heart rate. To use the table, find your age in the vertical column, and look at the corresponding pulse in the next column. To use the graph, find your age along the bottom line and trace a line straight up the graph. From that point trace a line horizontally to the vertical line, and the point of intersection is your target heart rate.

HOW TO TAKE YOUR PULSE

It's best to take the pulse at the radial artery in the wrist, using the middle finger. You'll find this artery on the thumb side of the wrist near the edge. Just touch the area—don't press, since you won't feel the pulse if you do.

Take the pulse for ten seconds only and then multiply this figure by six. This is your heart rate per minute. We don't take the pulse for one minute or even fifteen seconds, since the heart beat will slow down considerably during this time, making the result inaccurate.

DRINK WATER BEFORE YOU EXERCISE

This will replace the fluid you lose due to sweating and is especially important in summer. It is necessary to drink *before* you exercise because this helps to keep your body temperature from rising when exercising.

You should drink about two glasses of water. Don't drink sugar drinks, such as soft drinks and sports drinks, since sugar interferes with absorption of water.

Don't rely on thirst to warn you of dehydration. During strenuous exercise 'thirst sensors' in the throat lose sensitivity and can fail to send out 'drink' signals.

COOLING DOWN AFTER EXERCISE

Warming up before exercise is not essential, unless you are prone to injuries, since it is not strenuous activity. If you're training at an athletic standard, that's a different matter.

To cool down after the exercise, just slow down whatever you are doing for a few minutes. If you are doing brisk walking, for example, then just walk slowly for a few minutes.

It's especially important after jogging to walk for a few minutes. Jogging causes blood to accumulate in the legs and walking assists the body to return the blood to the rest of the body.

HOW WILL YOU KNOW WHEN YOU ARE FIT?

1 Your resting pulse rate will decrease, since your heart doesn't have to work as hard to pump the same amount of blood. After a few months your pulse should go down about ten beats. For example, if your resting

pulse rate is around the average of seventy beats per minute, it should reduce to around sixty beats per minute. Later it may go as low as fifty or less. When you are fit, your heart will beat around 15 million times per year less than the unfit person. This greatly reduces stress on the heart and is probably the main reason why you will live a lot longer than the unfit person.
2   You will feel less tired after exercise and during the rest of the day.
3   You will need to work a little harder during exercise to reach your target heart rate. But because you are fit, you will not feel you are working harder.

DON'T OVEREXERCISE

I cannot emphasise enough the fact that you should not overexercise.

Overexercise means:
- Pushing yourself too hard; that is, exceeding 80 per cent of your maximum pulse.
- Doing the same exercise more than three times a week if you are over thirty years old.

The results of overexercising are:
- Loss of protein, since protein is needed to provide energy and tissue repair. This will cause loss of muscle structure and weak muscles.
- Low energy level, since you are overtaxing your system.

If you wish to get fit fast, then exercise for longer periods.

WHAT IF YOU'RE SICK?

If you are suffering from some illness which involves the whole system, such as a cold, it's best not to exercise until you have recovered. This is because your body needs plenty of rest to maximise its recuperative powers.

I would advise a brisk walk for no longer than half an hour a day. This is much less strenuous than other exercises.

The Double Fat-Burning Exercises

IMPORTANT REMINDERS BEFORE YOU START

1 ● Frequency and Duration of Exercise

Until you have lost all the fat you require it is advisable to exercise six days a week. Once you have achieved your goal, say in three to six months, you can then maintain your fat loss by just exercising three times a week.

During the initial stage, if you are *under* thirty years old, you may do the double fat-burning exercises six days a week. If you are *over* thirty years old, you will need to do different exercises on alternate days. So, for three days a week do the double fat-burning exercises and on the three alternate days do some aerobic exercise such as jogging, walking, aerobics etc.

Regarding duration of exercise, for *optimum* results I recommend that you do the double fat-burning exercises for twenty minutes. Do each exercise for between one to two minutes and repeat the cycle two more times, so that total time is about twenty minutes.

When you do aerobic exercise, the duration depends on which one you do. These are the recommended times for the different types of exercises:
- Jogging—23 minutes
- Aerobics—23 minutes
- Walking—30 minutes
- Cycling—30 minutes
- Swimming—30 minutes

Don't forget you only have to do the additional three days of aerobic exercise until you have lost all the fat you want to. After that you can maintain that fat loss with just three days a week of the double fat-burning exercises.

Please remember not to weigh yourself to check your progress. Muscle is heavier than fat so, as your fat is replaced by lean muscle, you may not lose weight. The best indicators are measuring your waist, needing smaller size clothing and looking slimmer in the mirror. Of course, you will also feel much better.

2 • Intensity of Exercise

To find how hard you need to exercise, you just have to take your pulse after exercise. To take your pulse just put your middle finger lightly on the thumb side of your wrist near the edge. Take the pulse for ten seconds and then multiply this figure by six. This is your heart rate per minute.

You should aim for a pulse of 80 per cent of your maximum pulse (target heart rate). To find the target heart rate for your age just look up the table on page 52.

After a few weeks you'll know how hard to exercise to reach your target heart rate. Don't try to exercise harder than this—you'll do more harm than good.

3 • The Best Time To Exercise

Studies show that the greatest fat loss occurs with early evening exercise before the evening meal.

THE DOUBLE FAT-BURNING EXERCISES

All the following exercises stimulate muscle growth and are aerobic *at the same time*. When these two types of exercise are performed simultaneously they produce the double fat-burning results.

The best exercises to do are the five core exercises: skipping; sit-ups; push-ups; chair-stepping; and the rowing machine. The sit-ups and push-ups will need to be done quite quickly to produce an aerobic effect. Do the push-ups with the knees bent resting on the floor, since this makes it much easier and less strenuous than the traditional straight-leg method.

If you find a particular exercise too difficult to do just omit it or, preferably, try doing it for a short time and gradually increase the time as you become better. Make sure your total exercise time is still about twenty minutes.

I recommend that you commence the exercise program with skipping or chair-stepping because these exercises help you reach your target heart rate very quickly. Once you reach your target heart rate it is relatively easy to maintain it without exercising too hard.

The Program Can Be Done Without Equipment

Certain exercise equipment is useful because it is an easy way to produce muscle resistance. This form of exercise rapidly converts fat to muscle. Nevertheless, the program can be satisfactorily done without equipment.

If you wish to purchase just one piece of equipment, I would recommend a rowing machine (with universal joints), since this is excellent for developing the chest, bust, shoulder and arm muscles—areas often neglected with other exercise equipment such as exercise bikes and stepper type equipment.

THE FIVE CORE EXERCISES

Exercise 1: Skipping

Skipping is an excellent exercise both aerobically and from a muscle-stimulating point of view. It burns more kilojoules than any other exercise and strengthens muscles throughout the entire body. In addition, it reduces fat on legs, thighs and hips. Skipping ropes are very portable; you can take them anywhere and they don't cost much.

If you can afford to, pay a few extra dollars and buy a leather rope because they are heavier and go through the air faster.

If you find skipping or any other exercise difficult or inconvenient, you may omit it and spend extra time on the other exercises.

The best way to skip is to jump with both feet at once, picking up your feet just high enough for the rope to pass under. If you jump too high, you will cause jarring stress to the lower back. Wear good sports shoes with shock-absorbing material in them and skip on a thick mat or foam to prevent jarring stress.

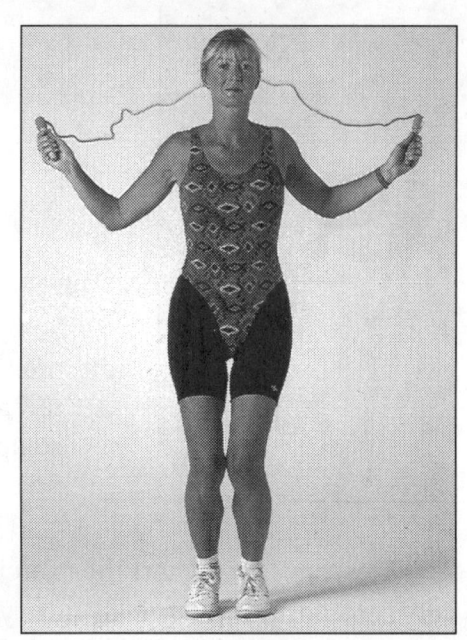

Exercise 2: Chair-stepping

This is a good indoor exercise; it's just as aerobic as skipping and doesn't have a jarring effect.

Just use an old chair and, if you're very unfit, start off with a low stool around fifteen centimetres high.

All you do is step up and down from the chair. Here is the best way to do it:

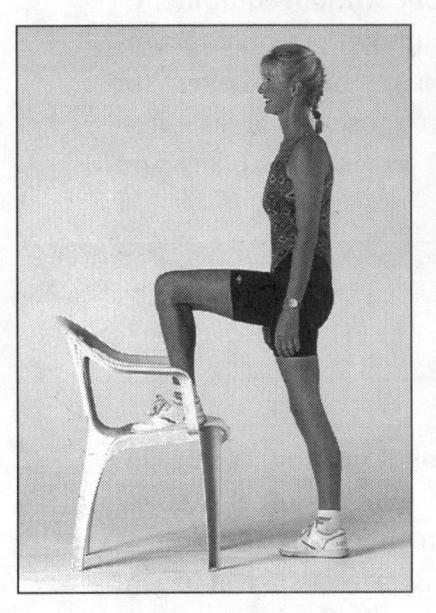

(a) Step on to the chair with the left foot.

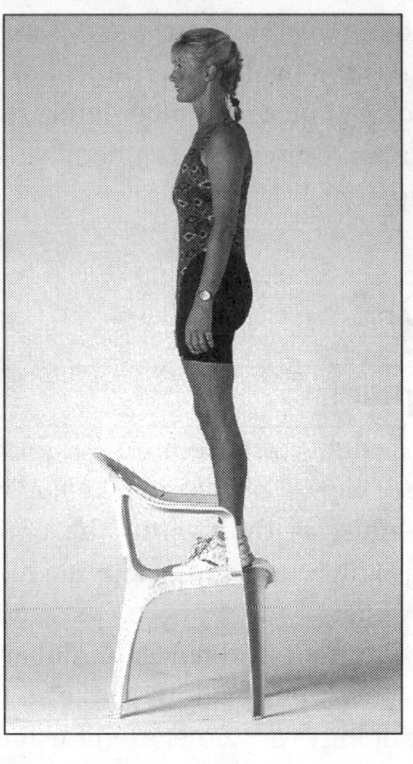

(b) Bring the right foot up too.

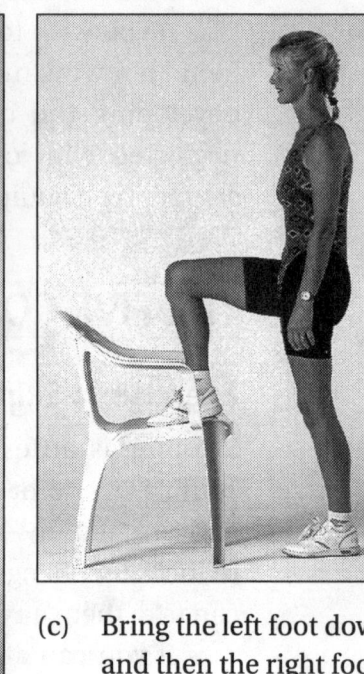

(c) Bring the left foot down and then the right foot.

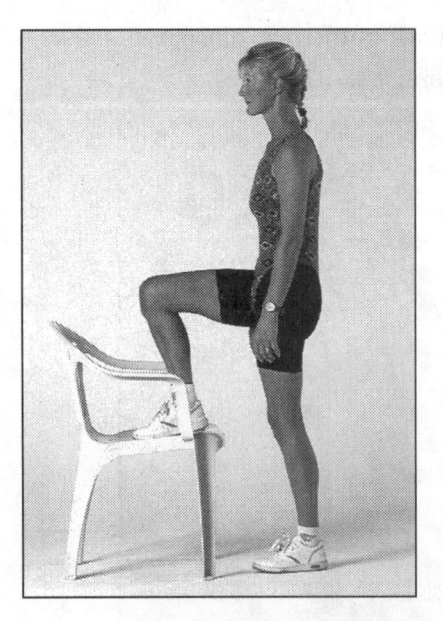

(d) After about one minute reverse the sequence by stepping on to the chair first with the right foot.

You may like to start the exercise program with chair-stepping as it is very aerobic and will quickly raise your heart rate to your target heart rate.

Exercise 3: Sit-ups

Lie on your back with your knees bent, anchoring your feet under a ledge of some kind. Place your hands behind your head. Lift your body to the sitting position using your stomach muscles.

Remember to do the sit-ups quite quickly to obtain an aerobic effect as well as a muscle-stimulating effect.

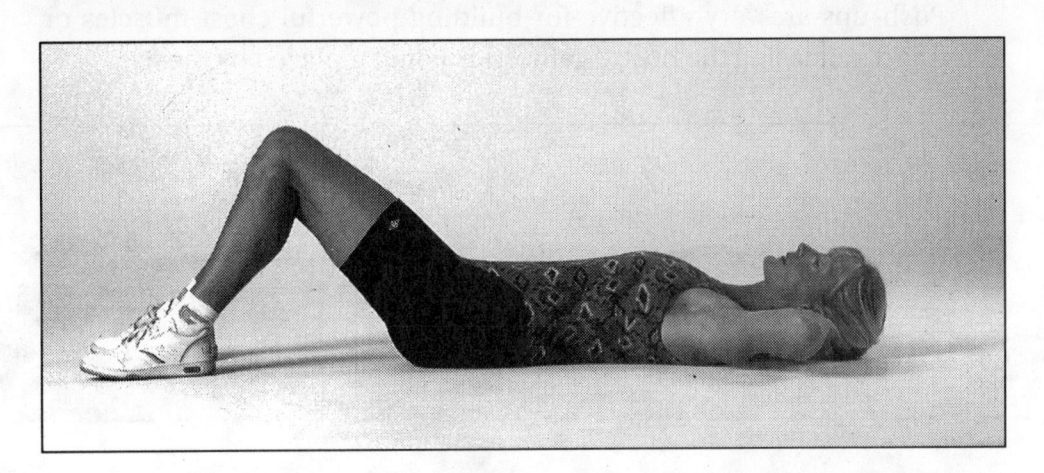

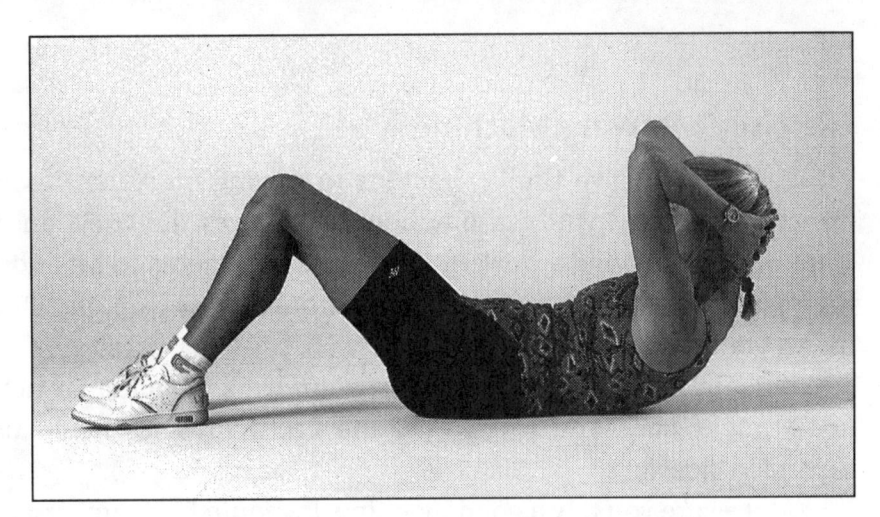

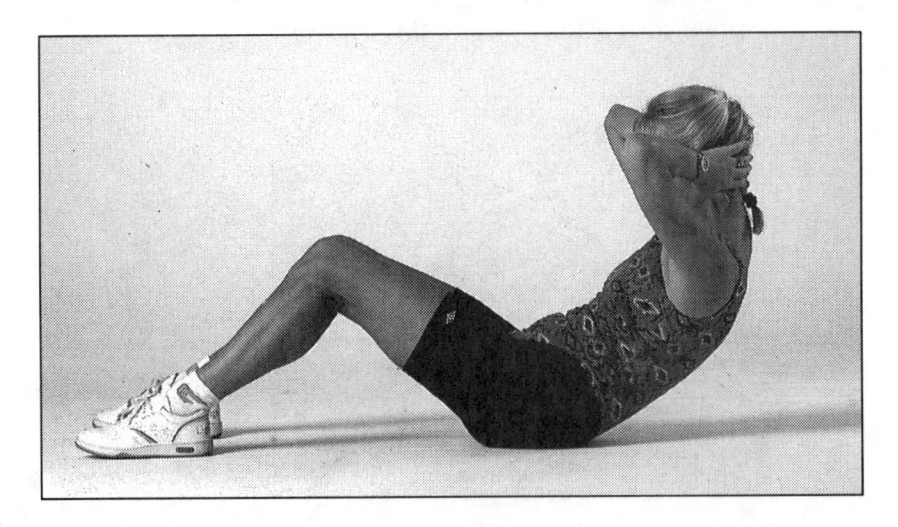

Exercise 4: Push-ups

For most people, the standard push-up would be too difficult to start with. To make them easier, instead of keeping your legs straight, rest your bent knees on the floor. Just raise and lower your body off the ground, using your arms. Keep your upper body straight. Start off with ten and work up to thirty over a few months.

Push-ups are very effective for building powerful chest muscles or lifting and increasing the bust. Again, fat is being replaced by muscle.

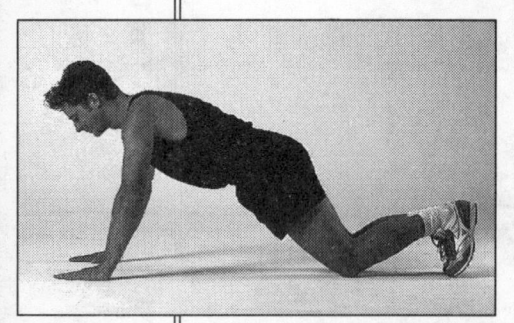

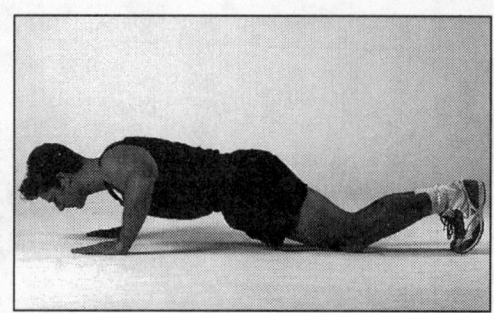

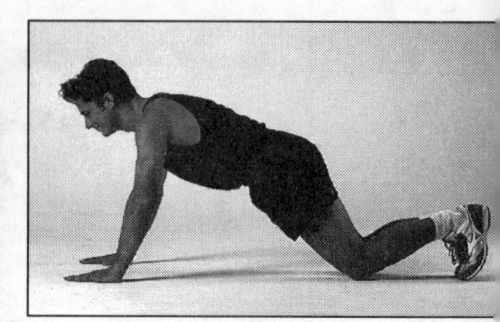

Exercise 5: Rowing Machine

These machines give similar benefits to rowing on water. It is the best exercise apparatus you can buy because it gives the chest an excellent work-out. It will build a powerful wide chest in men and lift and increase the bust size of women. It also gives the shoulders, arms, stomach, legs and back a good work-out.

To gain maximum benefit move your arms in a circular motion not just straight back and forth. Feel the chest muscles being used and expanded sideways.

Make sure you buy a good machine. It should have universal joints so you can move your arms in a circular motion.

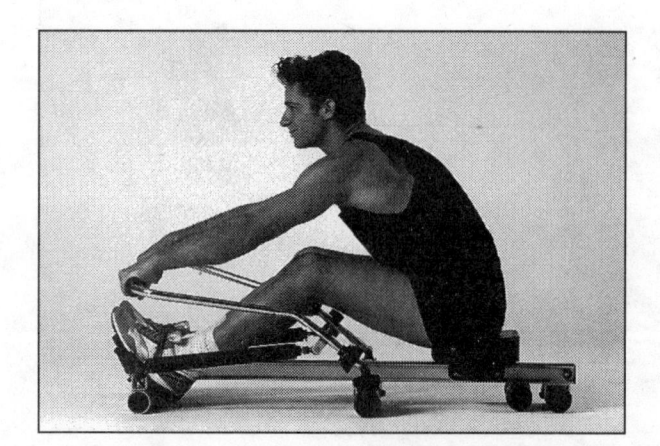

The Five-minute Super Fat Loss Exercises

THE SUPER FAT LOSS EXERCISES

If you wish to lose fat very quickly, you only have to do an extra five minutes a day of purely muscle-stimulating (strength) exercises. These are done very slowly with maximum resistance to stimulate muscle growth and replace even more fat in your body.

These exercises are very potent. They are the most effective muscle-stimulating exercises selected from Chinese kung fu, Indian yoga and Western body-building exercise systems. They also exercise every major muscle group in the body, resulting in a fine physique as well as fat loss.

You don't have to do all the exercises every day. For example, you could do the kung fu and yoga for three days a week and on three alternate days do the western body-building exercises. This way you will do all the exercises but spend only an extra five minutes a day.

If there is any particular exercise in this routine that you don't like or are not particularly good at, just omit it. It's not necessary to do all the exercises.

ANCIENT INDIAN BODY-BUILDING EXERCISES

As well as being very potent body-building exercises, these exercises will firm and tone up every major muscle group in your body. They will replace some of your fat with muscle and produce an increase in your metabolic rate.

These exercises should be done very slowly and if possible in front of a mirror so you can observe your movements.

Exercise 1: Weight Lifting

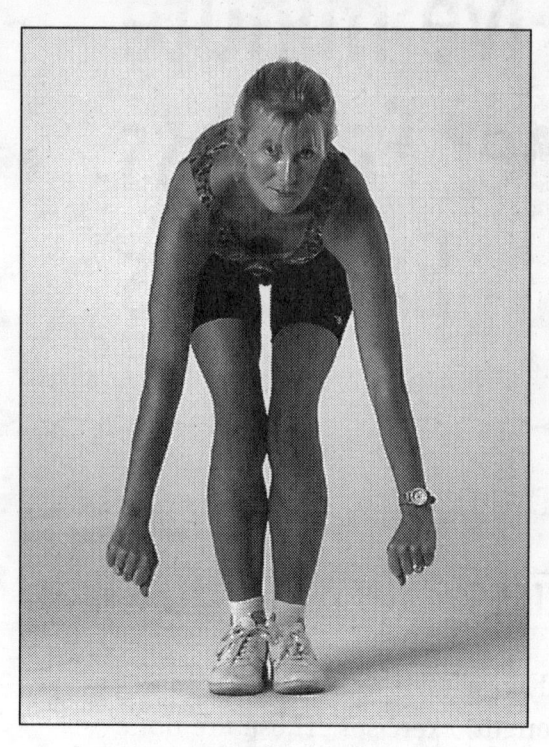

(a) Bend forward, grasp with both hands an imaginary heavy weight and snatch it up to shoulder height.

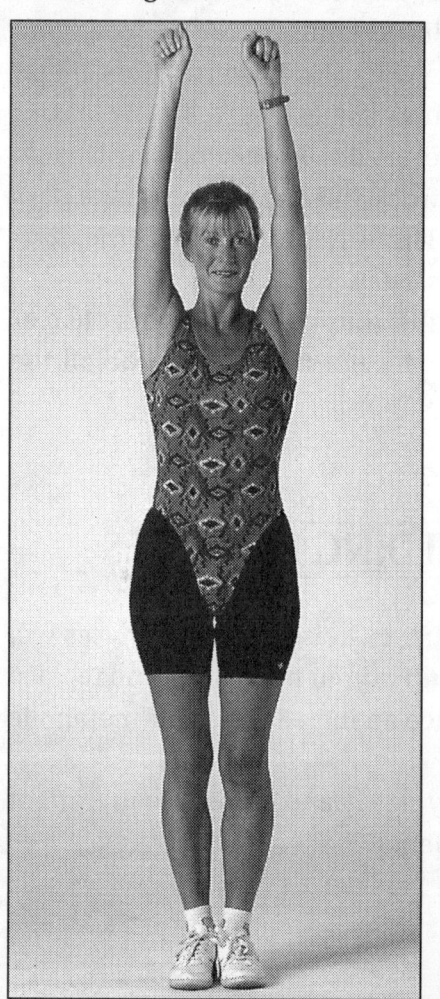

(b) Jump into the weight-lift stance—feet apart, flexing at the knees.

(c) Push the imaginary weight over your head with outstretched arms.

Remember to do the exercise in front of a mirror so you can watch your movements and perform the exercise so slowly that it takes about thirty seconds. Repeat once more.

Exercise 2: Swimming

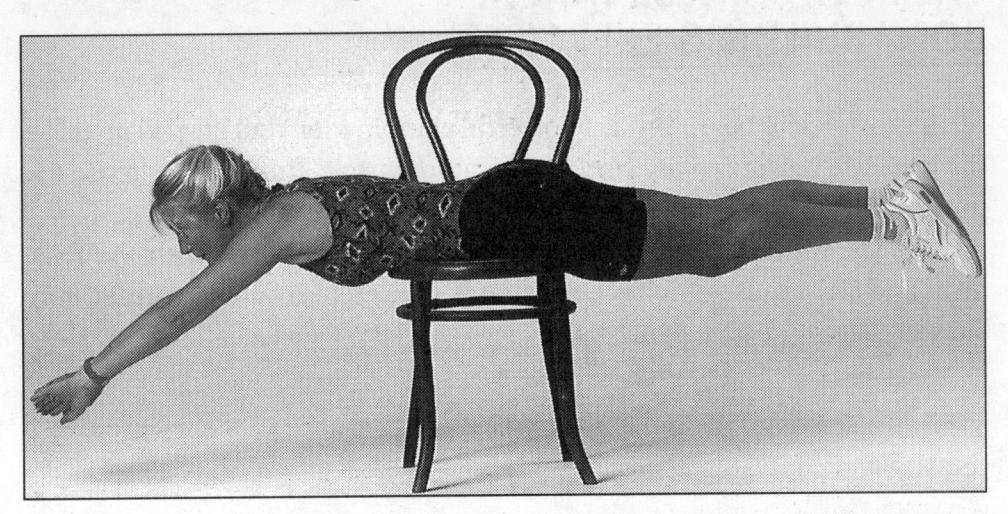

Lie on your stomach on a narrow bench or high stool and go through the motions of swimming—do both overarm (crawl) and breaststroke. Keep it up for about one minute.

Swimming is an excellent exercise, again exercising and developing all the major muscle groups. Now you can get the same benefit without the inconvenience of going to the swimming pool because you are holding your muscles in tension as you do these exercises, which has the same effect as the resistance from water when you swim in a pool.

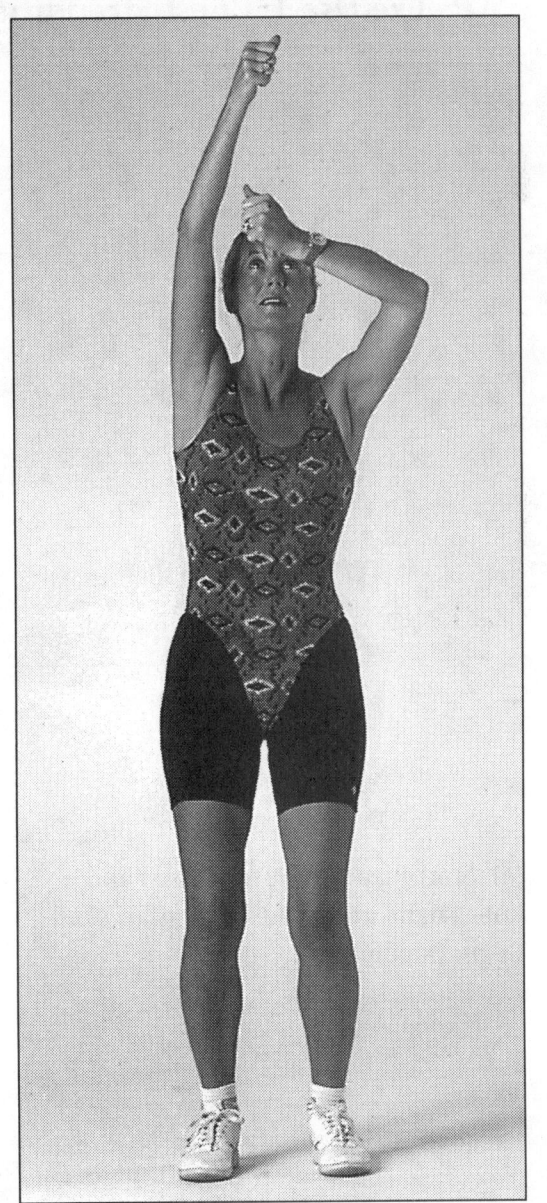

Exercise 3: Rope Climbing

Imagine that you are pulling down on a rope in order to climb it. Make sure you go through the motions slowly and keep your arm and chest muscles in tension. Keep going for about thirty seconds.

THE BEST CHINESE TAI CHI BODY-BUILDING EXERCISES

All three exercises below build a powerful chest in men and lift and increase the bust size in women. By converting fat to muscle, they also increase the metabolic rate of the whole body and hence burn up even more fat.

All the movements for these exercises must be done with the fists, arms and chest muscles in tension (that is, contracted) and performed very slowly.

Exercise 1: Chest Strengthener 1

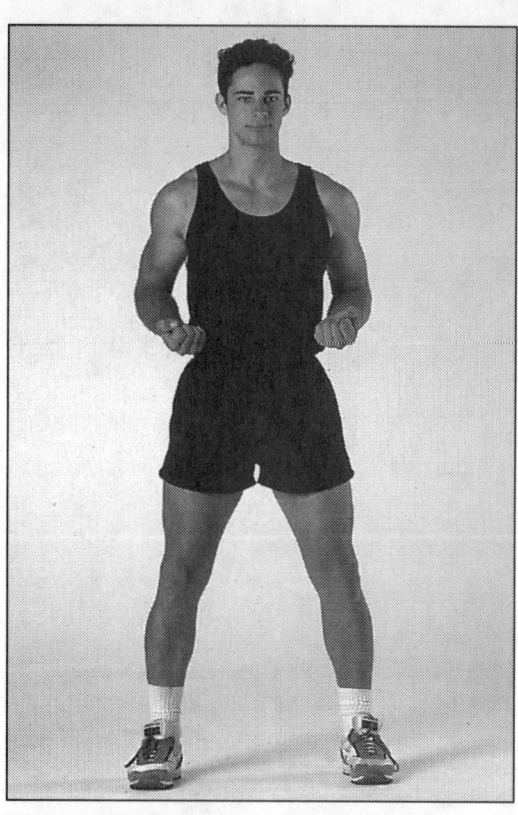

(a) Starting position: legs apart and knees bent, arms and fists tensed up. Begin inhaling.

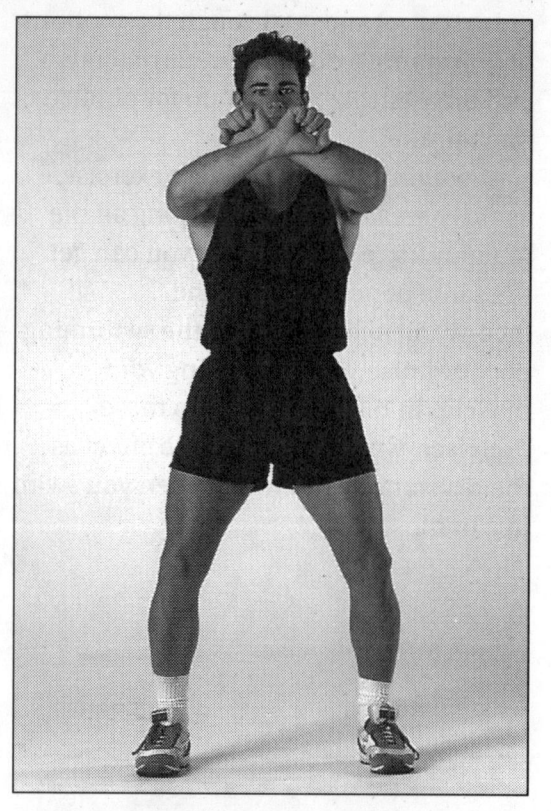

(b) Inhaling, bring your fists up in two intersecting arcs that cross in front of your face. If the exercise is being performed properly your upper arms should be parallel to the floor. From this point, the exercise is essentially a circular movement performed simultaneously with both arms, which inscribe two intersecting circles in the air.

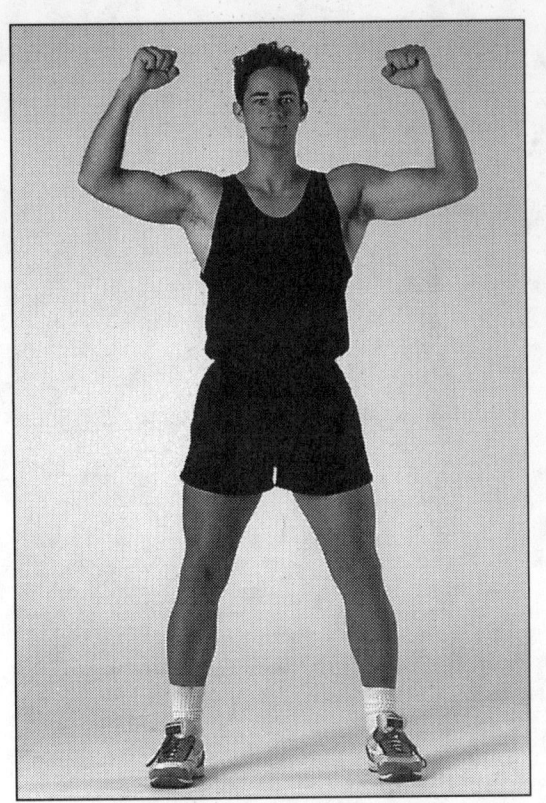

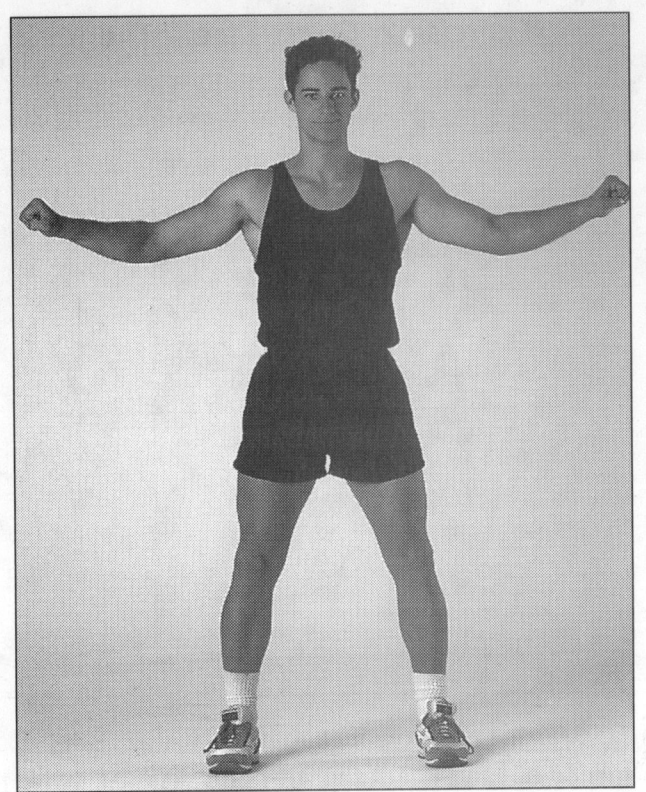

(c) Still inhaling, continue the arc your fists were making in the previous movement, until they are no longer intersecting and are above your head. Since your arms are moving in a circular fashion your elbows must be bent. Also note that up to this point the back of each hand is facing away from you; this will continue through one more movement and then will change.

(d) Exhaling, bring your fists down to eye level, keeping them on the same plane as the rest of your torso. Stay in this position until you have exhaled completely.

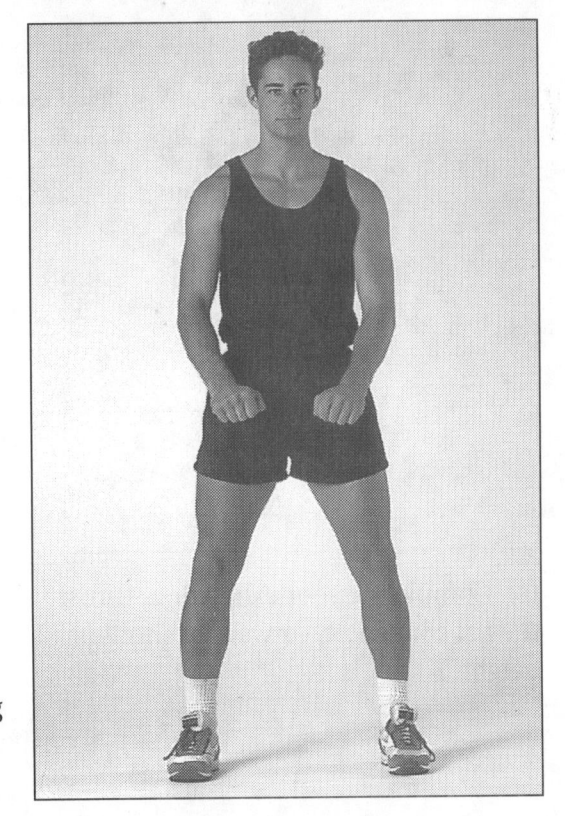

(e) Inhaling, turn your fists outward so that the backs of your hands are now uppermost. Then bring both arms downwards in front of your body, forming two circles that will once again intersect.
    Repeat two more times.

Exercise 2: Chest Strengthener 2

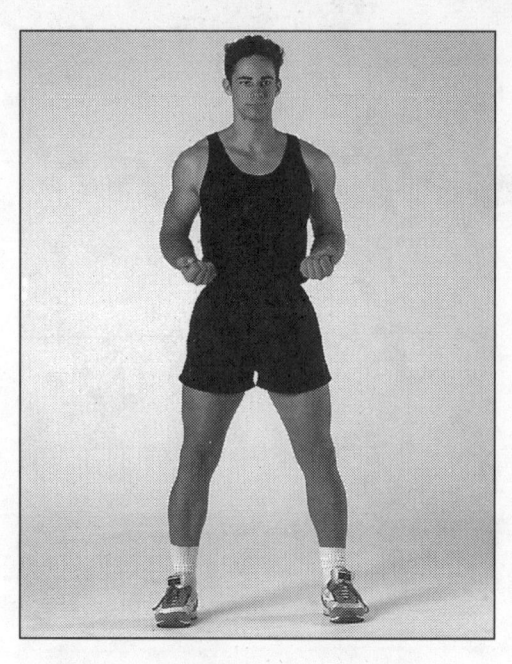

(a) Starting position: feet apart and turned out and knees slightly bent, fists by your side and elbows extended backwards slightly.

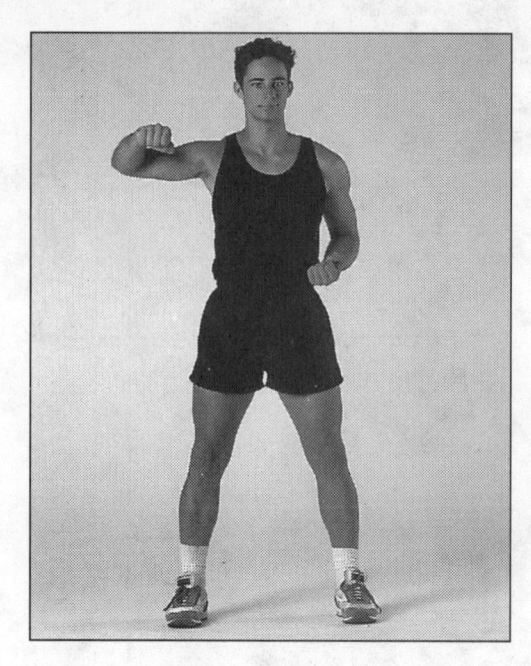

(b) Exhaling slowly, raise the elbow while turning the wrist.

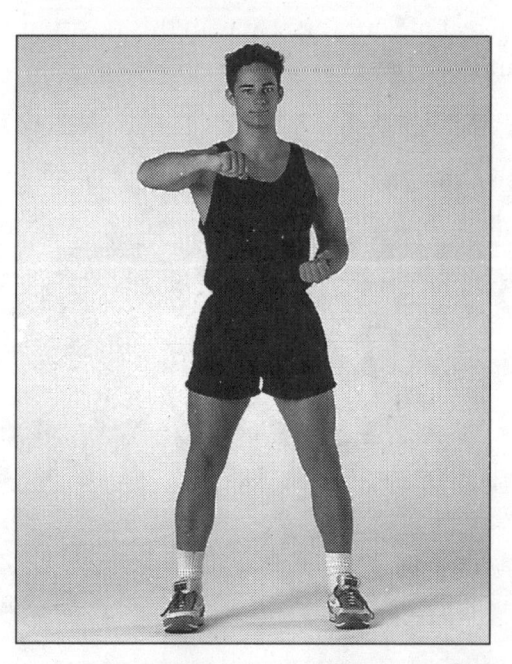

(c) Completing your exhalation, thrust the fist completely forward at shoulder height.

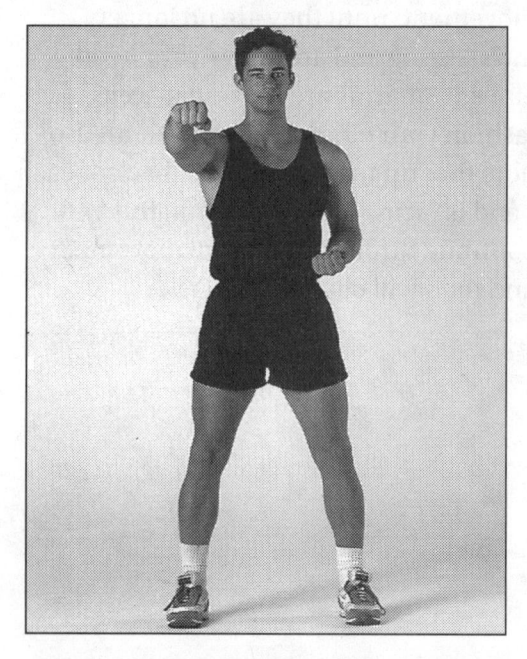

(d) Inhaling gradually bring the fist back to the side, following the same path that was covered when it was thrust out.

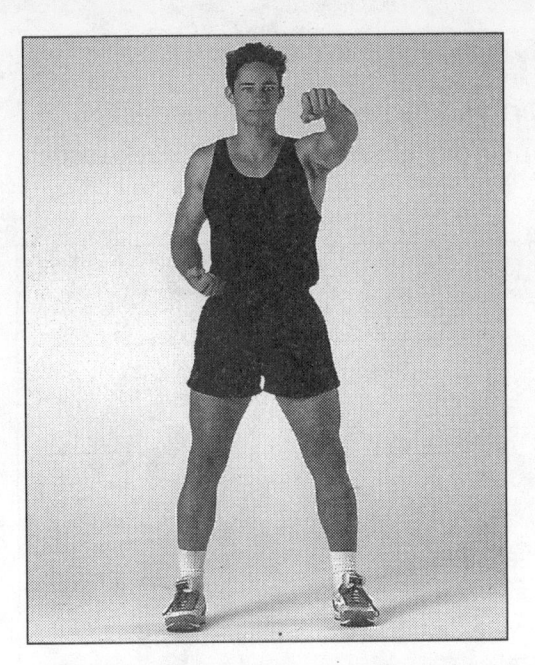

(e) Exhaling, make the left arm and fist follow the same movements as the right.
Inhale, return the left arm to the side.

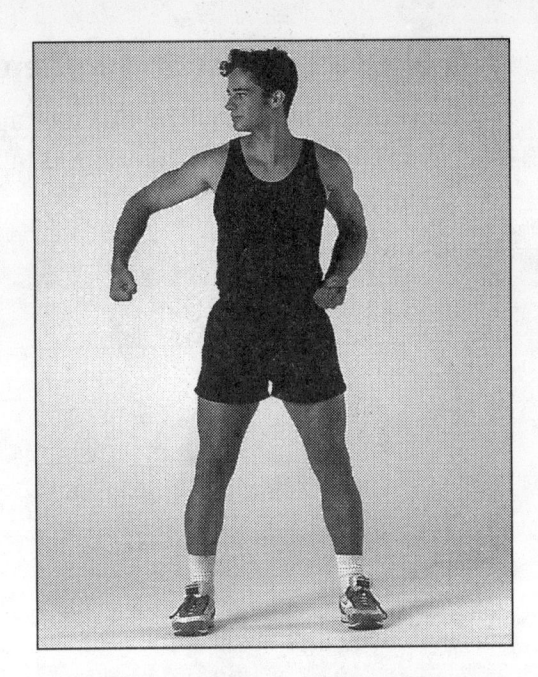

(f) Exhaling, raise the upper right arm and using the elbow as a pivotal point, gradually push out the forearm and the fist and keep them on the same plane as the torso.

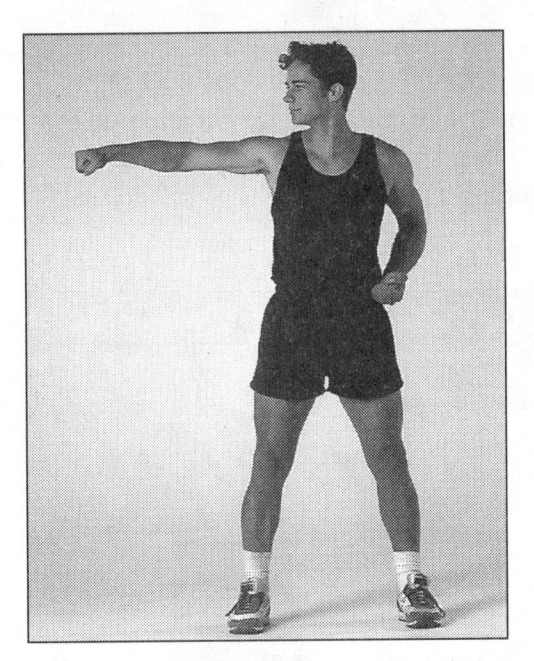

(g) Emptying your lungs completely, push out the right forearm and fist until the right arm is parallel to the floor and shoulder high.
Inhaling return the arm to the side, following the same movements that brought it out from the body.

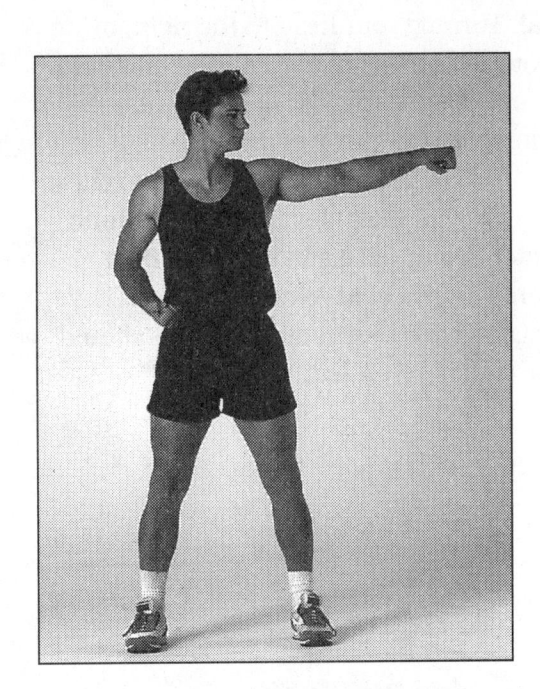

(h) Exhaling, push the left arm outward in an identical manner to the right.
Inhaling, return the left arm to the side. This completes one performance. Repeat once more.

Exercise 3: Chest Strengthener 3

Start this exercise with your feet apart and turned out and knees slightly bent. Hold your fists by your side and your elbows extended backwards slightly.

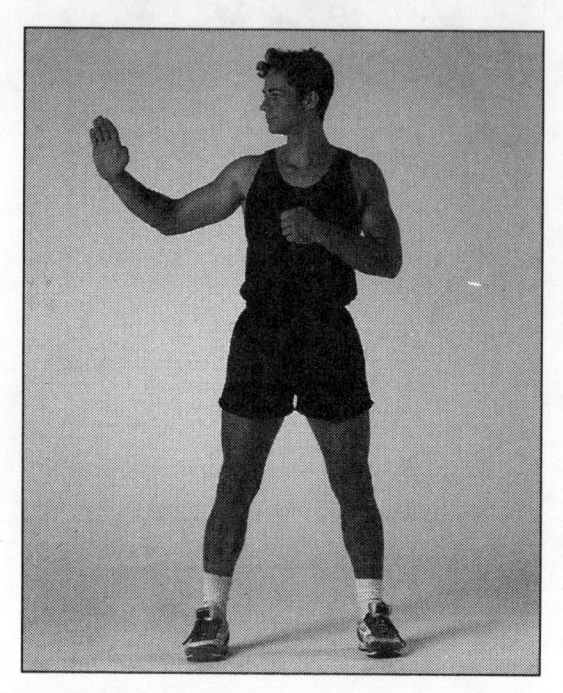

(a) Turning your head to the right, bring your left arm across your chest and hold it in a claw shape just as if you were clutching the string of a bow.

The right hand is brought up to chest height with the index finger and thumb extended upward and the remaining three fingers bent. When the hands have reached this position, your lungs should be completely filled.

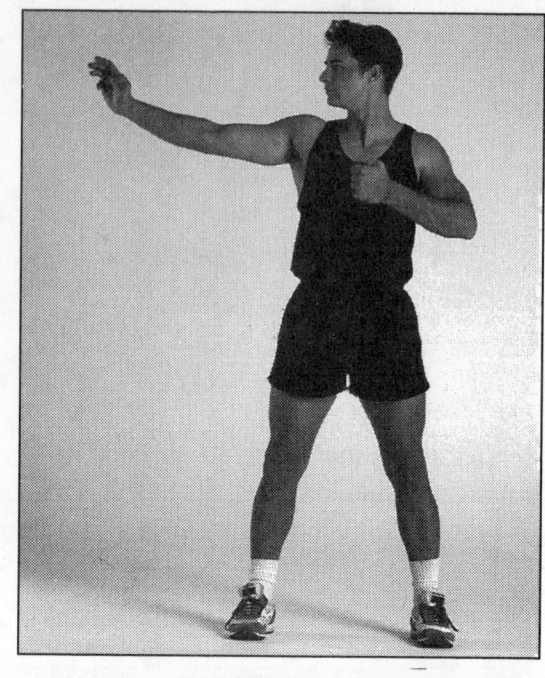

(b) Exhaling, gradually push the right hand out to shoulder height and pull the left hand back, almost as if you were pulling a real bow taut.

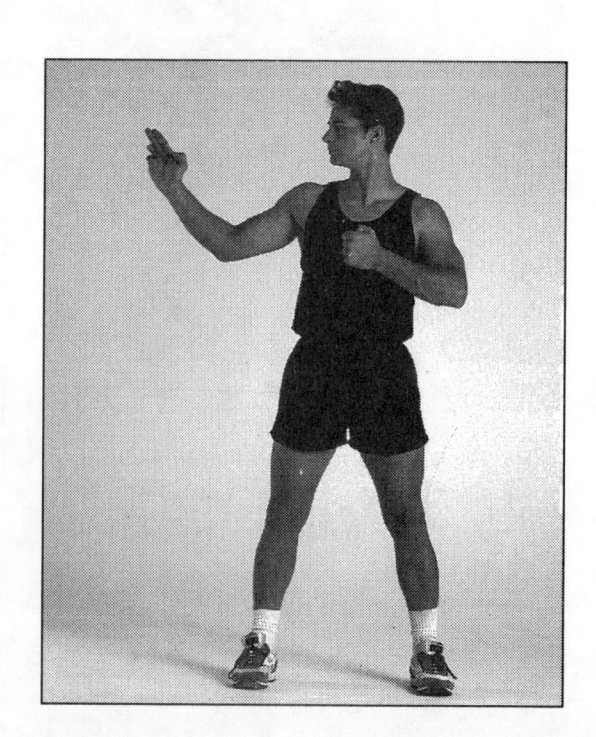

(c) After the maximum stretch point is reached, relax the bow while exhaling completely. Note how the hands gradually dissolve the bow's structure.

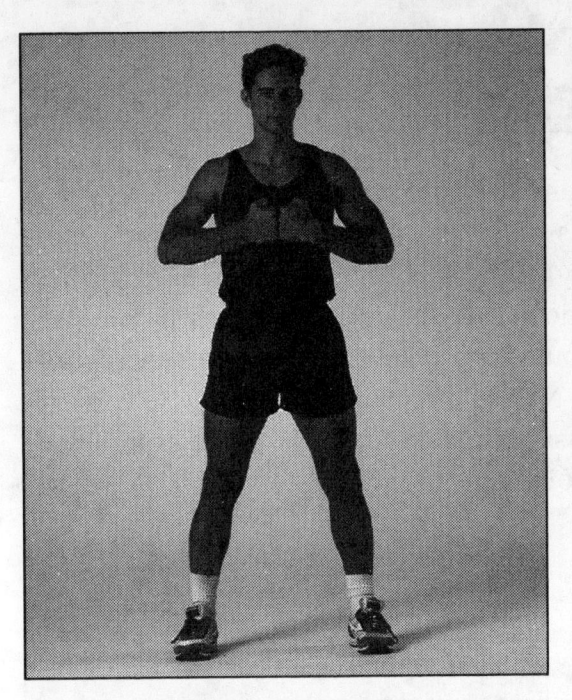

(d) The bow is dissolved completely as both hands pass in front of the chest and you begin a new cycle of inhalation.

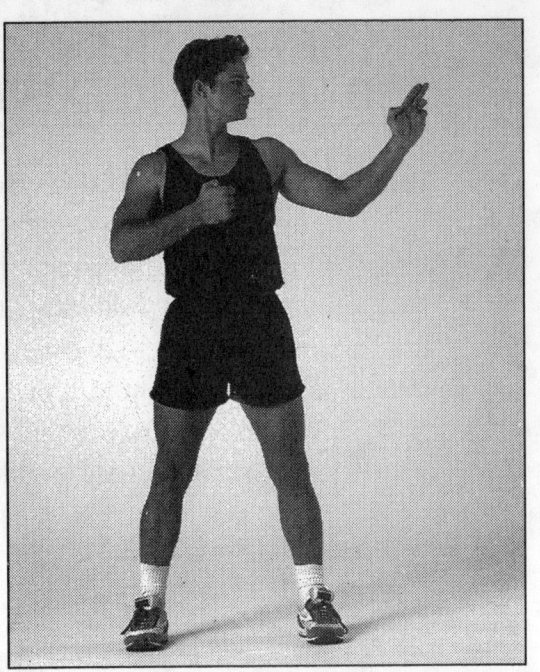

(e) Still inhaling, re-form the bow on the left side, with the right hand in the claw shape and the left as the energy focal point.

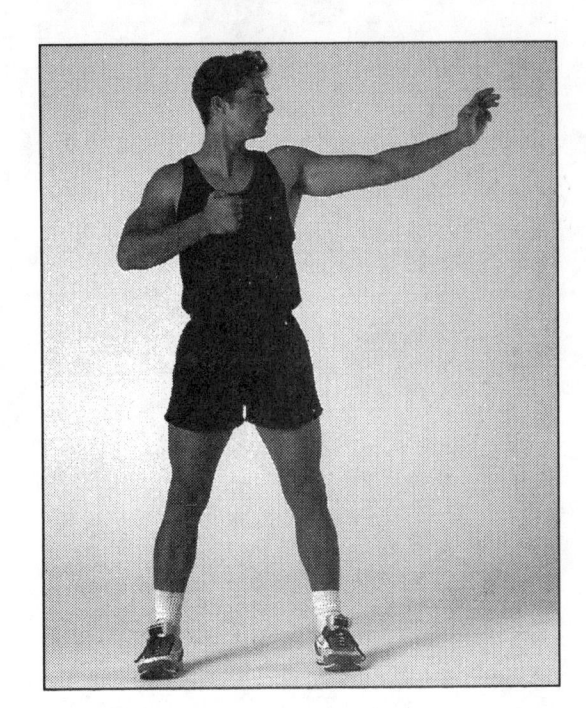

(f) Exhaling, pull the bow taut, as it was earlier on the right side of your body.
Still exhaling, relax the bow and return the hands to the original position.
Repeat once more.

THE BEST WESTERN BODY-BUILDING EXERCISES

Perform each movement slowly for maximum benefit.

For exercises using weights, start with the weight that you can manage. For women that is usually 1.5 to 2.25 kilograms; for men 2.25 to 4.5 kilograms. Do two to three repetitions without stopping. Inhale before you lift. Exhale and count to two as you raise a weight. Inhale again and count to four as you bring it back down. Never hold your breath.

Expect some muscle soreness for the first few days. If you experience pain, it's a sign that you are overdoing it.

Exercise 1: Lunge

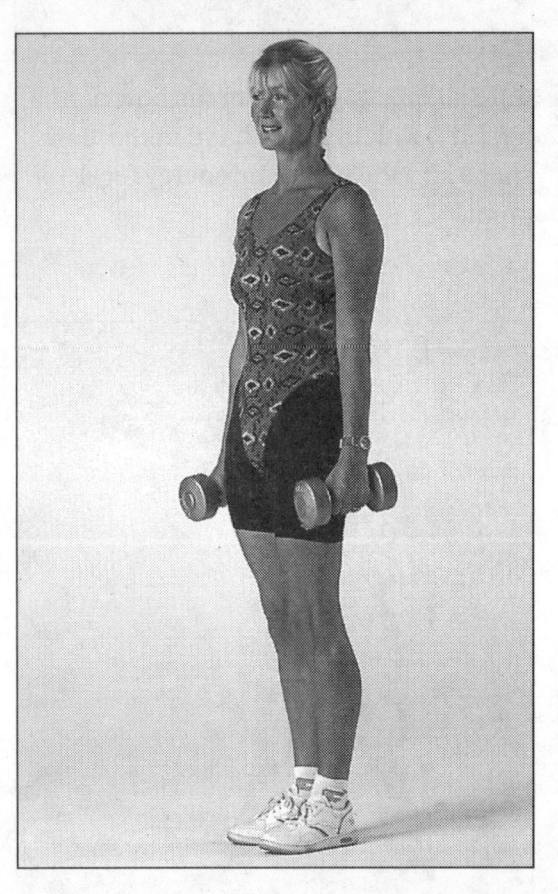

(a) Stand with feet together and a weight in each hand.

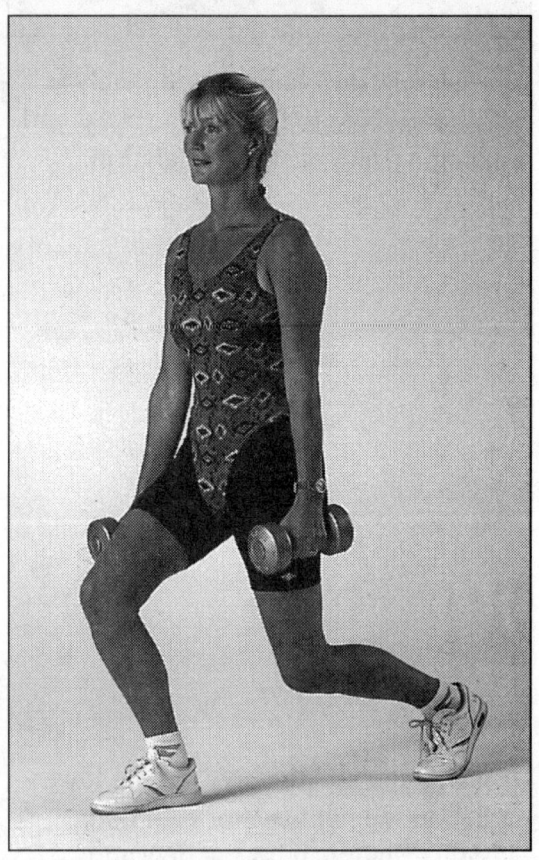

(b) Step forward with the right foot, knee bent directly over the foot. Left leg should be slightly flexed, with left foot on the floor.

Keeping the back straight, push body up again to starting position, using only your right leg. Repeat with left leg.

Exercise 2: Overhead Press

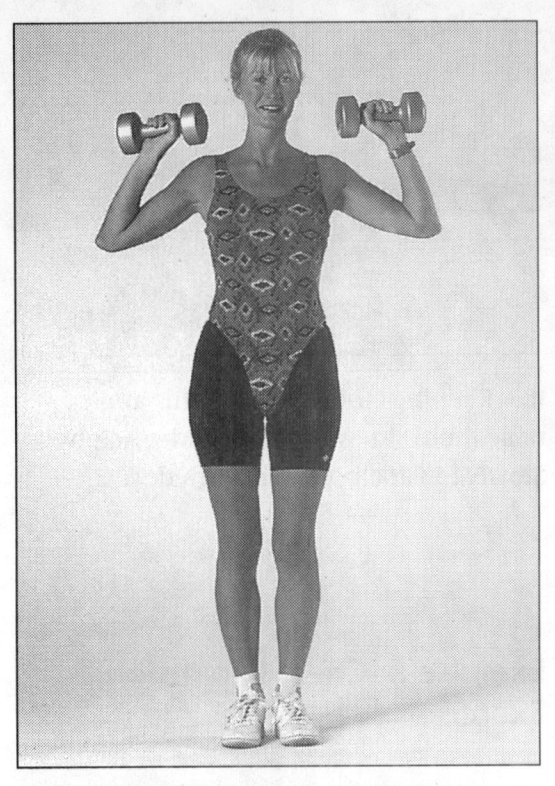

(a) You can do this exercise standing or sitting with your back against back of chair and feet on floor.

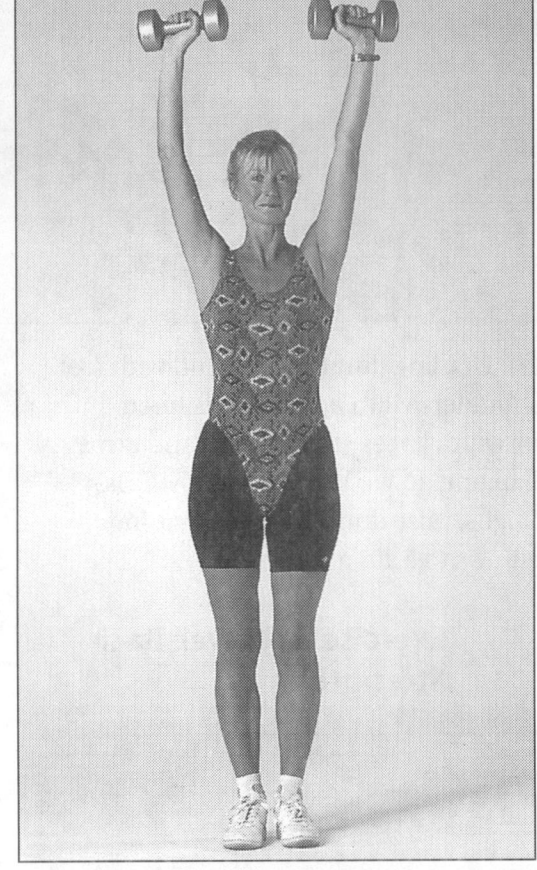

(b) With a dumbbell in each hand, palms forward, at shoulder level, slowly raise the dumbbells overhead, then lower them back to shoulder level.

Exercise 3: Triceps Extension

You can do this exercise either sitting or standing.
(a) Hold the dumbbells overhead with both hands, arms extended.

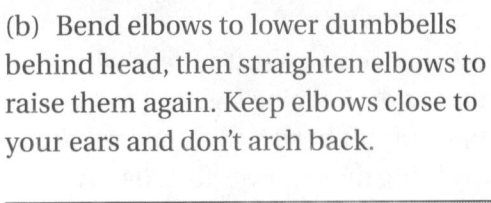

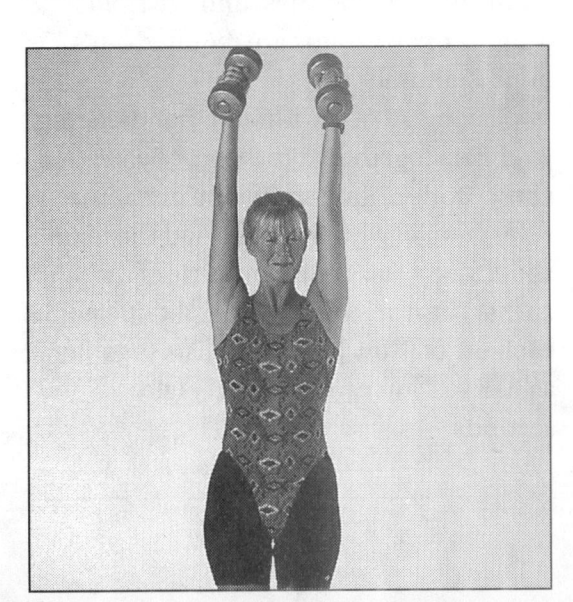

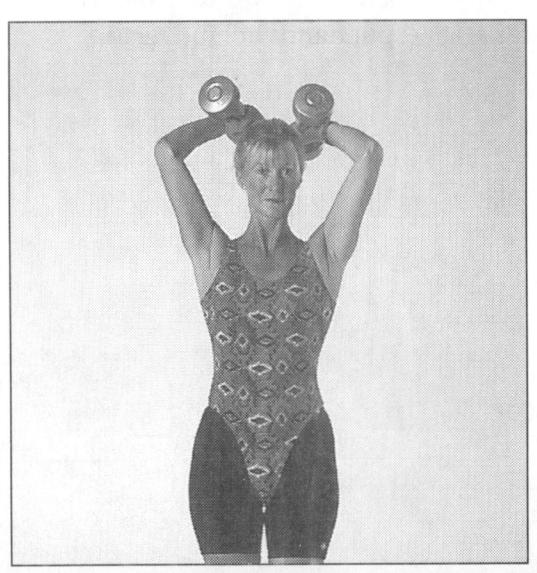

(b) Bend elbows to lower dumbbells behind head, then straighten elbows to raise them again. Keep elbows close to your ears and don't arch back.

Exercise 4: Lateral Raise

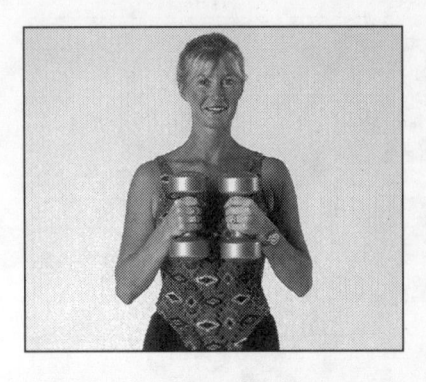

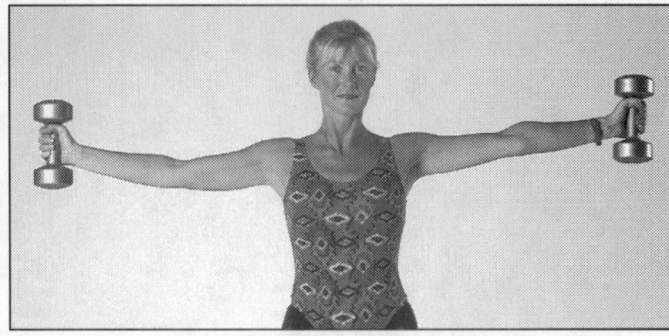

(a) Holding dumbbells, stand with feet shoulder-width apart, pelvis tilted forward, knees slightly bent and arms hanging down. With palms towards thighs, raise dumbbells by bending elbows to a 90° angle.

(b) Keeping elbows bent at this angle, raise them sideways to shoulder height. Slowly lower elbows back to sides.

Exercise 5: Lower Back Strengthener

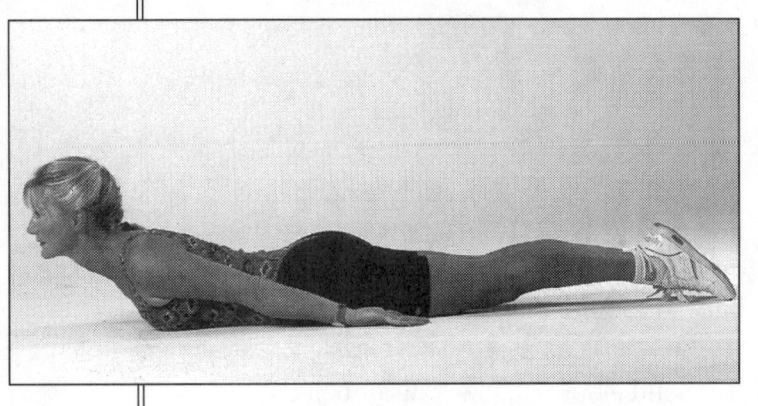

Lie on stomach on a soft surface with hands at side. Keeping legs and feet on floor, slowly lift head and shoulders, then slowly bring them down. To add more resistance, put hands behind head.

Exercise 6: Chest Expansion Exercise

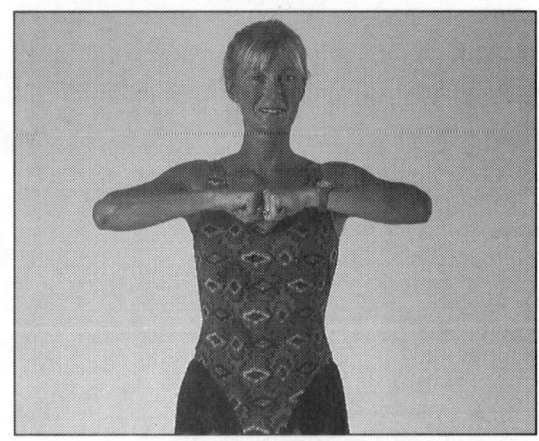

This is the most potent Western exercise for developing the chest and bust. No weights or apparatus are required—it's purely natural.

Just make fists with both hands. Bring your fists together at the level of your chest. Both elbows should be out at the side, parallel with the floor, and the fists should be a few centimetres from the chest. The arms are in a straight line with each other. Now push both fists together as hard as you can for about eight seconds.

Part Three

Eat Yourself Thin — The Nutritional Approach

The Nutritional Way to Quick and Permanent Fat Loss

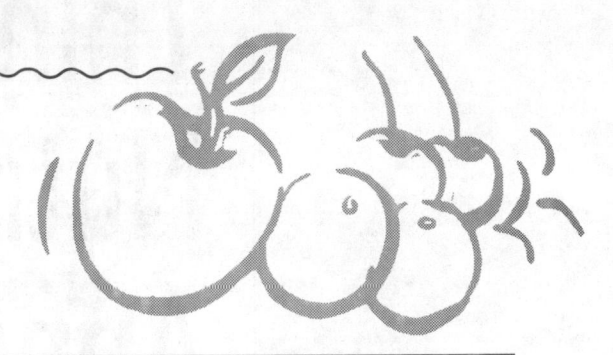

HOW A HIGH COMPLEX CARBOHYDRATE DIET CAUSES SLIMMING

Although dieting doesn't work (see pages 18–24), you nevertheless can lose additional fat by applying sound scientific nutritional principles and, at the same time, increase your health level.

The main nutritional guideline to follow is to replace some of your high fat/sugar foods with high complex carbohydrate foods such as fruits, wholegrains and vegetables. This is not dieting, since you are merely partially replacing one type of food with another type of food. In the process, you are taking in fewer kilojoules and increasing your health level. In short, to lose fat we don't need to eat less food, just different kinds of food. In the process, we are automatically taking in less fat and sugar without dieting or feeling hungry.

In practice, this substitution is very easily done, since by eating nutritious complex carbohydrates your appetite centre will be satisfied and you will feel no desire for eating extra sugar/fat foods. That is, you will start to lose fat automatically simply by slightly modifying your eating habits.

STUDIES CONFIRM THAT A HIGH COMPLEX CARBOHYDRATE DIET CAUSES FAT LOSS

One study done in 1976 proves the benefit of applying the above principle. Researchers fed a high fat diet to one group of rats and a high complex carbohydrate diet to another. The high fat group became about three times more efficient at storing fat. In another study, rats fed a high fat diet gained much more weight than a comparable group of rats fed a high-carbohydrate diet, even though the kilojoules in the two diets were the same.

Studies on humans show similar results to those on rats. One study on humans showed that people who ate high-carbohydrate meals tended to feel satisfied at half the calorie level of those who ate high fat meals.

The Chinese Are Living Proof

For practical evidence of the slimming effects of a high complex carbohydrate diet, we need to look no further than the diet of the Chinese. A Cornell University nutritional biochemist named T. Colin Campbell participated in a six-year long survey of the diet and health of 6500 Chinese subjects. He found that Chinese people eat about 20 per cent more kilojoules on the average than we do yet there's virtually no obesity in China.

According to Campbell, Chinese people do not become obese because they eat a plant-based diet full of carbohydrates and fibre but very low in fat and animal protein. They obtain on average 77 per cent of their kilojoules from carbohydrates and only 15 per cent of their kilojoules from fat. Australians and Americans consume an average of 45 per cent of kilojoules from carbohydrates and 39 per cent from fat.

The Chinese, with their high complex carbohydrate diet, not only have no obesity, they are also much healthier than western people. The average Chinese cholesterol level is 127, ours is 221. The heart disease rate in China is one-sixteenth of the US/Australian rate, and their rate for colon cancer is one-fifth of ours. As the Chinese move to a more western diet, their disease rate increases.

Research Evidence

When researchers fed rats high fat/sugar calorie diets, the rats grew tumours; when they fed them low-calorie complex carbohydrate foods, the tumours went away.

Conclusion

By eating a diet high in complex carbohydrates, you will increase your health level and, as an extra bonus, become slimmer. This nutritious diet will make you feel satisfied and therefore prevent bingeing and sneaking between meals, a major cause of weight increase.

HOW EATING NUTRITIOUS FOODS CAUSES LOSS OF FAT

Nutritious foods are fresh, high-nutrient foods such as fruits, vegetables, whole grains, raw nuts, soya milk and fish. Raw food is the most nourishing food since none of the nutrients have been destroyed by cooking. Good examples of raw food to include in your diet are fruits, salad, raw nuts and bean sprouts (see also below).

Nutritious foods cause the body to shed fat via three mechanisms.

1. When you start eating more nutritious foods you will obviously replace some of the processed foods you've been accustomed to eating. Since processed food is much higher in fat or sugar content than nourishing food, you are now consuming considerably fewer kilojoules.
2. The appetite centre in the brain is programmed to register satisfaction when the body has taken in sufficient nutrients and bulk (fibre). Nutritious food is far higher in nutrient and fibre content than processed food and so your body is satisfied with a smaller quantity of nutritious food than processed food.
3. The increased fibre content of nutritious food causes fat loss in three ways. First, as explained above, consumption of bulky food is registered on the appetite centre of the brain more quickly than non-fibrous food. Second, fibrous food holds water and thus creates even more bulk which fills up your stomach and makes you feel satisfied. Third, a stomach full of sticky soluble fibre such as porridge (oatmeal), empties more slowly, prolonging the time until you feel hungry again.

RAW FOOD

Up to 70 per cent of your diet should be raw food: fruit; salad; sprouts; and raw nuts. This is very easy to achieve by having some fruit at breakfast-time, and fruit and nuts for morning/afternoon tea and snacks. Include salad and sprouts (alfalfa and mung beans) with your lunch or evening meal. You are merely replacing some of your cooked and processed foods with raw foods.

Enzymes, the life of food, are only present in raw, unprocessed foods. Cooking, canning and processing of food destroys the enzymes in the food. The pasteurisation of milk also destroys the enzymes in milk and actually makes milk detrimental to health. Pasteurisation (heating) changes the chemical structure of the protein (casein) and sugar (lactose) in milk and makes it difficult to digest for most people. In strict moderation no harm is done. My recommendation is soya milk but not everybody likes soya milk or can afford it. Skim milk is the second choice.

How Raw Food Makes You Slim

There are several reasons why a 70 per cent raw food diet will cause you to lose excess fat. These reasons are as follows:

- Since raw food is very nourishing, your body needs less food to meet its nutrient requirements. This results in a reduction in appetite.
- Raw food is low in fat and sugar and therefore low in kilojoules.
- The high nutrient content of raw food causes your body, including your digestive system, to work more efficiently leading to more efficient metabolism of fat.
- Raw food does not create toxins in the digestive system. This means the digestive system is more efficient at assimilating nutrients and therefore, less food is required. This again results in reduced appetite.

Other Benefits of Raw Food

High Vitality Level
Your vitality is enhanced because enzymes and vitamins are not being destroyed by heating and processing.

Reverses Ageing
- Skin—becomes tighter. This results in less wrinkles and a natural lift to the face.
- Eyes—become brighter and clearer.
- Hair—becomes thicker and shinier. Grey hair starts to regain its natural colour.
- Lifespan—increases.

Improvement In Brain Function
Since the brain is better nourished, our thinking becomes clearer, our memory improves, and we become calmer.

Another advantage of a 70 per cent raw diet is that it solves most of our other dietary problems. It means your diet must be low in fat, protein and sugar, since raw food is low in these items.

Wild animals, eating only raw food, do not get sick. Put these animals in the zoo and give them cooked, processed food, and they will become sick. Some communities, such as the Hunzas in northern Pakistan and certain African tribes who eat mostly raw food, do not get the degenerative diseases of civilisation.

Fibre and Slimming

What Is Fibre?
The term 'dietary fibre' refers to the parts of plants that pass through the human stomach and small intestine undigested —ranging from the brittle husks of whole wheat to the stringy pods of green beans. There are two principal types: soluble and insoluble.

Soluble Fibre When soluble fibre reaches the colon (large intestine), bacteria breaks it down into fatty acids that can be absorbed. Two common types of soluble fibre are pectins (found in apples, oranges and other fruits) and gums (found in foods such as oat bran and barley).

Insoluble Fibre Insoluble fibre is not broken down by bacteria in the colon. All fibrous foods contain some insoluble fibre, but the most concentrated supply is found in corn and wheat bran. Whole grains and lentils are also rich sources.

A balance of soluble and insoluble fibre gives digesting food a soft and bulky consistency, helping to move it at a steady pace—neither too fast nor too slow—through the digestive tract.

How Fibre Causes Fat Loss
Foods high in fibre (fruits, vegetables and whole grain products) create a bulky feeling in the stomach. This full feeling is relayed to the brain and causes a reduction in appetite.

To dramatically increase this fullness feeling, drink a glass of water with high fibre foods. The water causes the fibre to swell and this increased bulk results in a further reduction in appetite. Practical examples of this are drinking a glass of water with a wholemeal sandwich, a banana milkshake, wholemeal cereal and milk.

One of the reasons why fruit is so effective for slimming is due to its high fibre content mixed with its own mineral-rich fluid.

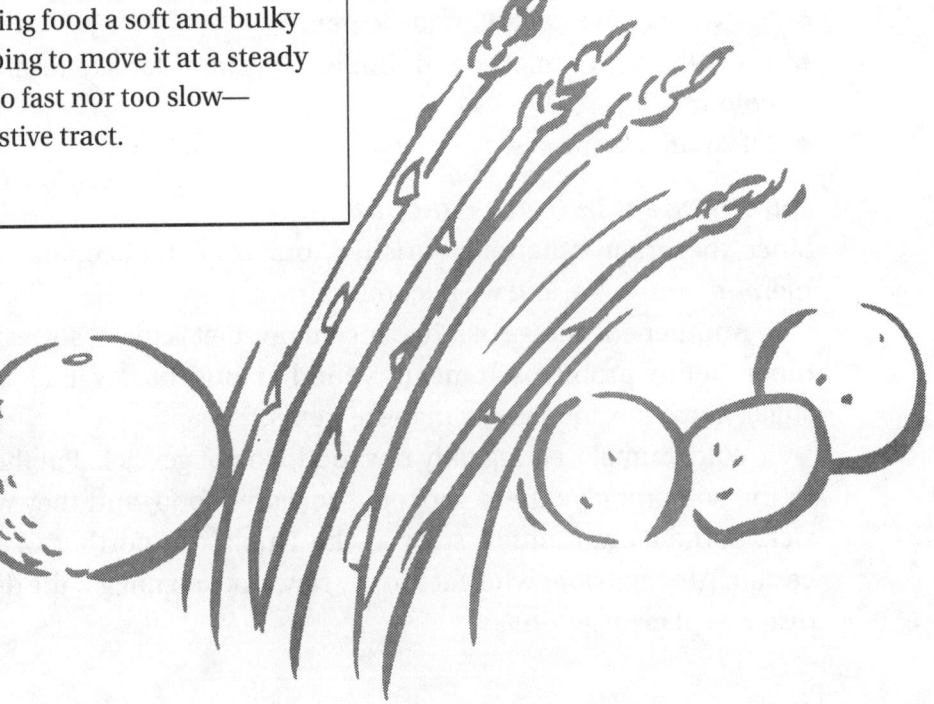

Other Health Benefits of Fibre

- Fibre reduces your cholesterol level. It does this by mechanically and chemically removing cholesterol from your intestines. The fibre in soya beans and oat bran is especially effective in reducing cholesterol.
- Fibre reduces your blood pressure.
- Fibre causes a reduction in heart disease because cholesterol and blood pressure levels are reduced. Countries which have high fibre diets have much lower rates of heart disease. Japan, which has the highest fibre diet of all nations, has only one-seventh the rate of heart attacks of the United States. Americans, like people in most other western countries, have a very low fibre diet, mainly due to eating refined carbohydrates and a lot of meat.
- Fibre is necessary for bowel regularity and has been shown to help prevent cancer of the colon.
- Fibre helps to regulate your blood sugar levels. It does this by helping to control the rate of absorption of glucose into the bloodstream. This prevents mood swings and helps in the treatment of obesity and diabetes.

The Best Sources of Fibre

All unrefined complex carbohydrates are good sources of fibre. This includes fruit, vegetables, whole grains such as wholemeal bread and cereals, and beans (lentils, chick peas). There is no need to put bran on your foods—just include plenty of the above foods in your diet. This way you're getting fibre in the correct proportion to other nutrients, and also eating nutritious food.

It's especially important not to give bran to young children. Young children need lots of calories and nutrients for growth. Too much fibre can cause them to feel full before they eat enough calories and nutrients for normal growth and development.

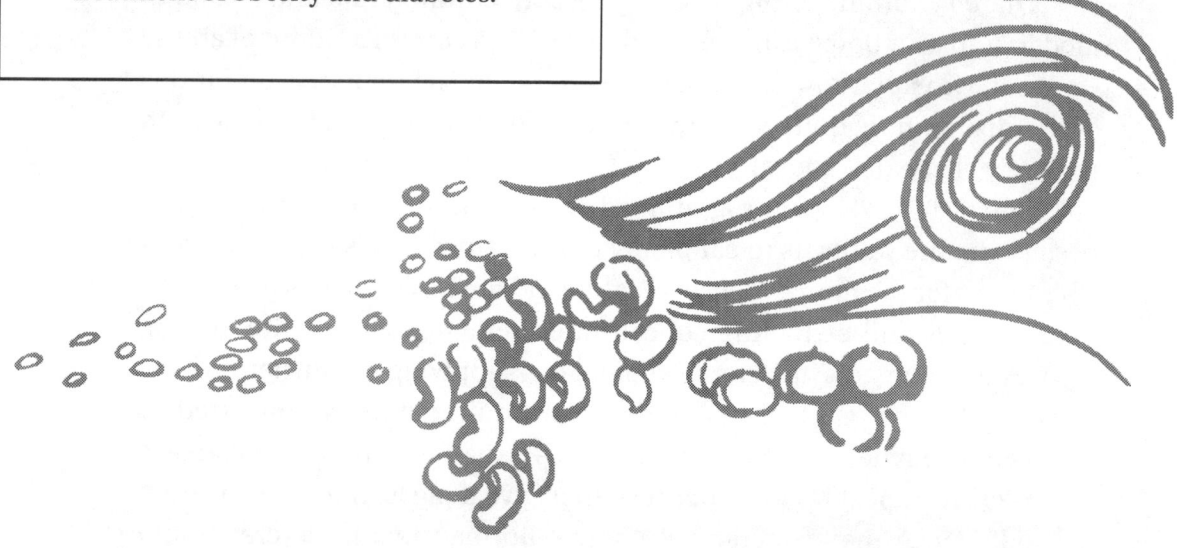

CONCENTRATED SUGARS AND FATS—
A MAJOR CAUSE OF WEIGHT PROBLEMS

The most concentrated kilojoules are found in fats and sugars. Different fats and sugars are essential for health but problems occur because we consume far too much. It is easy to eat too much fat and sugar because we eat it in concentrated forms.

Keep in mind even though you are reducing fats and sugars, you are not dieting. A whole chapter has already been devoted to showing how dieting doesn't work and ultimately makes you fatter. What you are doing is reducing unnatural processed foods and replacing them with natural fresh nourishing foods. There may be no reduction in the volume of food you eat but there will certainly be a reduction in the amount of kilojoules you are taking in. This is because fats and sugars are very kilojoule dense, that is, they contain a lot more kilojoules per gram than other foods.

Why Concentrated Fats and Sugars Cause Problems

Concentrated sugars (refined sugar) and concentrated fats (butter, cheese), are really processed foods which is not a natural state for food to be in. Milk does not exist as butter or cheese in nature. The fat in milk is extracted to make butter and cheese and so these products are actually processed, unnatural foods. The same applies to sugar. The natural form in which to eat sugar is the whole sugar cane or sugar beet. In this way, we obtain fibre and nutrients as well as the sugar. In addition, because we are eating a lot of fibre, we feel full very quickly, making it impossible to consume too much sugar.

There is nothing wrong with eating concentrated fats and sugars in moderation. Our bodies are designed to handle a certain amount of abuse! However, we eat far too much of these products. The main reason for this over-consumption, quite simply, is because they taste good (and are both relatively cheap nowadays).

Our taste buds are programmed to like the taste of sugar. This is because nature wants us to eat plenty of fruit, since this is the most nourishing food for the human species. Nature did not anticipate us processing natural foods and extracting concentrated refined sugar (white, brown, raw). Refined sugar is just empty kilojoules—supplying no nutrients to the body. Any sugar in excess of the body's requirements is converted to triglyceride (a type of fat) and stored as fat—usually in the stomach area.

Fats are appealing to us because they give a pleasant creamy texture to food. Hence the attraction of cheese, butter, cream, ice-cream and chocolate etc. Again, nature intended us to enjoy the small amounts of fat present in all natural foods; nature did not intend us to extract the fat and eat it on its own. Nature intended us to drink milk, not the concentrated fat of butter or cheese. Similarly, nature intended us to eat corn and olives, but not use the concentrated fat extractions of corn oil and olive oil for frying food.

Our bodies are simply not designed and have not evolved to handle concentrated sugars and fats. Our bodies are designed to function correctly on the whole food. That way we are getting complex carbohydrates and fibre as well as the fat content. For your car to operate efficiently, you fill it up with the correct petrol. You don't extract one chemical from the petrol and fill your car with that. Your car might still work but at much reduced efficiency and it certainly won't last as long. It's exactly the same with the human body. We can still operate on concentrated fats and sugars but not so efficiently. Throughout our lives our health will be impaired until, eventually, we get a disease such as heart disease (excess fat), or diabetes (excess sugar). We will age prematurely and die younger. And don't forget that while we are still alive, or at least just ticking over, we will be overweight.

You can see we pay a high price for eating too much concentrated fat and sugar. These products are so concentrated that you only have to eat a small amount to be eating a lot. Of course, the average person eats a lot of concentrated fat and sugar, so you can imagine the problems they are creating.

In addition, refined sugar causes obesity for the following reasons:
- The body converts excess sugar into fat.
- Sugar is such a taste tempter that people easily overeat when sweets are readily available.
- Sugar provides no bulk to warn the body that it has consumed a lot of kilojoules.
- Sugar has no nutrients so you still feel hungry after eating concentrated sugar foods.

ALL KILOJOULES AREN'T CREATED EQUAL

The latest research shows that eating high-fat and high-sugar foods, or those high in both sugar and fat, will make you gain more weight than if you eat a low-fat, low-sugar diet containing the same amount of kilojoules. This happens because the body uses up more energy to process carbohydrates than it does to assimilate fats. Also, only 3 per cent of dietary fat is burned during digestion, transport and storage—the rest is converted to body fat.

Fatty foods, such as chocolate, slip into our system almost effortlessly, whereas the body has to work quite hard to digest complex carbohydrates such as fruits and vegetables. A lot of energy is expended to digest these carbohydrates (about 10 per cent of the total kilojoules), which means there is less fat left in the body.

In other words, high fat/sugar foods are doubly bad for you. Not only are these foods the most kilojoule-laden foods, but their kilojoules have a greater weight-producing effect than kilojoules from other foods.

A study carried out at the University of Illinois, Chicago, observed overweight women who followed a high-fat diet (37 per cent fat kilojoules) for four weeks then a low-fat diet (only 20 per cent of fat kilojoules) for twenty weeks. Total body weight, lean body weight and fat weight were measured at the end of the high-fat period and at the end of the low-fat period.

It was found that the women lost weight during the low-fat diet period, despite consuming 19 per cent more kilojoules than they consumed on the high-fat diet. In addition to this, fat weight decreased 11.3 per cent and lean body weight increased 2.2 per cent. The researchers concluded that the fat content of the diet, not just the kilojoules, is an important consideration when designing weight loss programs.

FAT: ENEMY NUMBER ONE

Every gram of fat has 37 kilojoules which is more than double the amount carbohydrates and proteins have per gram. A tablespoon of margarine has 600 kilojoules and a tablespoon of oil has 740 kilojoules: you should be very moderate with these two products.

Try to adopt the non-fat habit. Wrap foods in foil, then grill or barbecue them instead of frying. Remember that fat not only makes you fat, but also clogs up your arteries making you a candidate for heart disease, high blood pressure, a stroke, diabetes and some types of cancer.

FAT CONTENT OF COMMON FOODS

Many of the foods we commonly eat are high in fat, as you probably realise. For example:

Butter and margarine	–	100% fat
Coconut and palm oil	–	86% fat
Cooking oil	–	100% fat

Cream cheese	–	90% fat
Mayonnaise	–	99.8% fat
Peanut butter	–	75% fat
Tartar sauce	–	95% fat

In comparison, most vegetables contain less than 10 per cent fat. A baked potato is only 1 per cent fat, but add two parts of butter and it increases to over 40 per cent. Most fruits contain less than 5 per cent fat.

- 30 grams of vegetables – 42 kilojoules
- 30 grams of oil – 940 kilojoules
  - ➡ You can eat about 25 grams of vegetables for every gram of fat.
  - ➡ You can eat 5 grams of fruit for every gram of sugar.
  - ➡ Ten roasted peanuts has the same amount of fat as 2.5 kilograms of potatoes.

Now can you see the reason for filling up on low-kilojoule nutritious food?

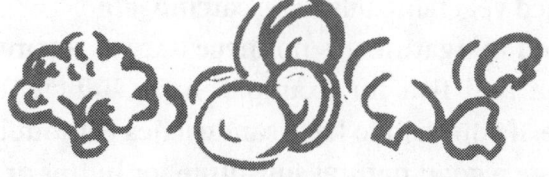

DO YOU HAVE A FAT TOOTH? (FAT ADDICTION)

Research at the Monell Chemical Senses Centre in Philadelphia has shown that we can have a fat tooth in the same way as we can have a sweet tooth. More importantly, the research also showed that this fat addiction can be broken.

Scientists experimented with three groups of people: one group ate a 'normal' generally high-fat diet; the second was instructed to adhere to a fat-restricted diet; and a third used low-fat substitutes for fatty food in a normal diet. The groups were tested and the pleasure ratings (degree of approval) of the range of foods was recorded during the twelve weeks they were on the diet and again twelve weeks after the cessation of the program.

At the end of the initial period, the researchers found a decrease in the pleasure ratings for fatty foods in the two groups with restricted fat intake. They also noticed a decrease in overall kilojoule intake and a decrease in body weight in these groups compared to the normal diet group.

At the end of the post-test period (twelve weeks later), the intake of fats and expressed satisfaction for fatty foods was still low in the low-fat diet group but not in the group using low-fat replacement foods.

The indication from this is that while fats may be addictive and help increase the total kilojoule intake in the diet, restricted use can break the addictiveness and quickly restore body weight equilibrium. Low-fat substitutes are not as effective as a low fat intake.

HOW TO REDUCE FAT

It's important to remember that all fats, whether saturated (meat, butter) or unsaturated (vegetable oils), have the same high kilojoule level.

Reduce Oil When Frying
Use a non-stick frying pan and heat the pan before adding the oil—you will need use a lot less oil this way.

Reduce Butter and Margarine
Both are very fattening. Don't be fooled thinking margarine is better for slimming. Margarine contains vegetable oils which are 100 per cent fat, just the same as the animal fat in butter. Health-wise you are better off with butter. Margarine contains vegetable oils which have been heated to very high temperatures and treated with chemicals. Some research has shown these processed vegetable oils to be carcinogenic.

Butter and margarine are not necessary as a spread on bread. Most meat, chicken and fish for example, have sufficient fat to produce a pleasant taste. If you wish to have sandwiches without meat/fish, bananas or avocados are a good natural substitute for butter or margarine. In fact, just plain banana sandwiches are very tasty.

Cheese
Buy low-fat varieties. Cottage cheese and ricotta cheese are low in fat.

Reduce Meat
The main problem with animal-derived protein is the high ratio of fat that comes with it. Fat represents over 80 per cent of the kilojoules in hot dogs, 65 per cent in hamburgers and about 50 per cent in fried chicken eaten with skin. Red meats and processed meats are also high in fat.

To reduce your fat intake, buy lean cuts and trim the visible fat off the meat before you cook it.

To help reduce your meat intake, don't make meat the main focus of the meal, but rather a condiment or complement to vegetables or grains, such as pasta or rice. You can cut the meat into small pieces or slices and combine it with lots of vegetables, and then stir fry, or make a soup or casserole.

Try to eat more fish and less meat. Fish has less fat and contains omega-3 oils, which lower your cholesterol levels. Fish is also very nutritious.

Buy Low-fat Foods
These days you can buy low-fat yoghurt, ice-cream, salad dressing, spreads and packeted frozen fish, etc.

Eat More Low-fat Foods

Eat plenty of fruit, vegetables and whole grains. These foods are very nourishing, and leave you too full to be tempted by high-fat foods.

Low-fat substitutes

Instead of:	Substitute:	Your Savings	
		Fat (grams)	Kilojoules
1 cup whole milk	1 cup skim milk	8	265
3 strips bacon	1 slice lean bacon	7	275
30 g potato chips	30 g low-salt pretzels	9	155
30 g cream cheese	30 g Neufchatel cheese	3	100
1 apple turnover	1 medium apple	14	730
½ cup sour cream	½ cup low-fat yoghurt	18	570
30 ml hot fudge sauce	30 ml chocolate syrup	4	134
1 cheeseburger with bacon	1 plain burger	16	920
90 g French fries	1 medium baked potato	14	220
30 g cheddar cheese	30 g skim mozzarella	5	175

OVERCOMING FAT-LOSS PLATEAUX

What Causes Fat-loss Plateaux?

Anyone who has tried to lose fat knows the frustration of hitting a 'plateau'—the point at which no further fat loss seems to be occurring even though diet is under control and you're exercising.

Plateaux are entirely natural in any loss of body mass. They are the result of the body adapting to changing energy demands and may last for a period of days, weeks, or even months.

A plateau may occur as the body becomes more 'efficient' in managing the restrictions that have been put on it. For example, for anybody exercising using the same routine for a long period, efficiency in carrying it out is improved and consequently the energy required (i.e. kilojoules used up) decreases.

Your food intake is affected in a similar way. Metabolism, like anything, gets better with practice, so the energy required for digestion of a particular food is likely to decrease as that food becomes more familiar.

The Solution

Plateaux can be countered by attacking the cause, that is, improved efficiency. In terms of exercise load, this means making exercise less efficient by changing:

- *Intensity*—increase the speed at which the exercise is performed.
- *Duration*—exercise for longer periods.
- *Frequency*—exercise more regularly, for example by adding 'incidental' exercise, such as walking upstairs instead of taking the elevator.
- *Type*—varying walking with cycling, swimming, aerobics.

With food intake as the other side of the energy equation, plateaux can be countered by:

- *Decreasing fat/sugar kilojoule intake*—but only where this is still high.
- *Increasing complex carbohydrate kilojoule intake*—where these kilojoules are too low.
- *Changing food type*—eating foods the body is not familiar with.

HOW TO REDUCE YOUR SUGAR INTAKE

Excess sugar (this includes alcohol), is stored as a type of fat called triglyceride. To bring your triglyceride level down, try to adopt the following measures.

- Replace sugar-sweetened soft drinks and fruit drinks with unsweetened fruit juice.
- Replace snacks and desserts such as cakes, biscuits and ice-cream with fruit.
- Replace cereals containing sugar with sugar-free cereals.
- Use sugar alternatives such as honey, molasses, dried fruit and fructose.
- Reduce alcohol by replacing some of it with mineral or soda water.

REDUCING FAT AND SUGAR IS NOT DIETING

Dieting implies cutting kilojoules across the board by reducing consumption of all food types (protein, carbohydrates and fats). However, protein and complex carbohydrates are usually not the problem. The problem is excess fat and sugar. In fact, when you start reducing protein and complex carbohydrate foods (bread, potatoes), the body's metabolism will slow down, including your capacity to burn fat.

To make matters worse, your slowed-down metabolism stays with you after you've resumed normal eating. It takes time and correct exercise to speed your metabolism up again.

This program simply replaces some of the excess fat/sugar foods you have been eating with nutritious foods.

We consume far too much fat and sugar. By reducing your fat and sugar intake, you are merely bringing your fat and sugar levels down to normal levels. This is not dieting.

THE IMPORTANCE OF BREAKFAST FOR SLIMMING

It's very important not to skip breakfast. Eating breakfast causes your metabolism to speed up for the whole day and, consequently, you burn up more calories.

One study showed that when people skipped breakfast, and consumed all their food at lunch and the evening meal, their metabolic rate decreased by 4.8 per cent. This would cause a weight increase of up to 2.5 kilograms a year.

I suggest you have both fruit and cereal for breakfast, preferably fruit first and then cereal about half an hour to one hour later.

The early morning fruit helps you to slim. It takes advantage of the body's natural food cycle. Between 4 a.m. and noon, the body eliminates a lot of its toxins (the eliminative cycle). This cycle promotes slimming in two ways. First, it helps remove the toxins stored in fat and muscle tissue—this reduces the general bulk of the body. Second, less toxins in the body means better digestion of the food you eat—this means more of the fat in your diet is broken down to produce energy instead of being stored as fat.

THE IMPORTANCE OF FRUIT FOR SLIMMING

In addition to a fruit breakfast being beneficial for slimming, fruit at any time of the day will encourage fat loss. This is mainly due to the fact that fruit is low in calories, yet high in nourishment. You only need to eat a small amount of fruit for the appetite centre in the brain to be satisfied.

HEALTHY SNACKS ASSIST SLIMMING

Medical research suggests that snacking helps with weight problems and generally makes you healthier when it is done correctly.

In a recent study at America's Cornell University, thirteen women ate as much as they wanted of forty-one low-fat foods for snacks and meals. In eleven weeks they lost an average of 2.5 kilograms.

A Canadian study by Dr David Jenkins, Professor of Medicine and Nutritional Sciences at the University of Toronto, produced even more unexpected results. For two-week periods, seven men ate the same healthy foods. During one period, they ate regular meals of breakfast, lunch and dinner. In the other part of the test, they ate the same foods divided into seventeen mini-meals. When researchers tested the men's blood they found the nibbling diet, in addition to causing fat loss, also lowered cholesterol levels by 8.5 per cent.

These findings show that large, infrequent meals supply more kilojoules than you require for the complex mechanisms that regulate the digestive and metabolic processes: thus the body does not use all the food as energy and the excess must be stored as fat. When you eat small meals the food is absorbed at a slow and steady rate, and there is little or no excess food left to be stored as fat.

The Best Snacks

The best snacks are those which are high in nutrition and low in fats. This includes fruits, carrots, air-popped popcorn, raw nuts, low-fat yoghurt and banana smoothies (no sugar or ice-cream).

The Best Time To Snack

Eat when you feel hungry, not at any specific time. Your body will let you know when to eat.

Four to six hours after you eat the liver depletes its store of carbohydrates. Your body needs these carbohydrates to convert to blood sugar. When your supply runs out you will feel a little tired and hungry. You may even get a headache. To keep energy high during the day, try not to go more than four hours without a snack.

A recent nutritional study suggests that an afternoon snack also improves brainpower. Researchers analysed the mental skills of eight students who ate a high-energy afternoon snack, then compared their performance after they switched to a caffeine-free diet soft drink. When the students snacked, they did 20 to 30 per cent better on memory and concentration tests.

Check Snack Food Labels

If you decide to snack from packets of food, you'll need to read the labels carefully. For example, if you read 'only 800 kilojoules', check to see if that is the total, or 800 kilojoules per serve, or per 100 grams. Be wary of gimmicks. A product labelled 'light' doesn't necessarily have a low kilojoule count. It could be lighter in colour, texture, taste, or contain marginally less fat than the regular product. Snacks advertised as 'cholesterol free' aren't always fat free. Cholesterol-free products contain no animal fat but may contain vegetable fat.

THE IMPORTANCE OF NOT OVEREATING

Why Overeating Is Harmful

- Food which is in excess of the body's requirements is not broken down properly and acts like a poison in the body.
- Excess food overtaxes the digestive system. This eventually reduces the efficiency of the digestive system and ultimately reduces the amount of nourishment you receive from all the food you eat.
- Overeating wastes your body's vital energy. Even with a moderate diet, digestion uses up around 10 per cent of your energy level. If you overeat, you can expend up to 60 per cent of your body's energy supply.
- Overeating causes fatigue and adversely affects mental clarity because most of your energy supply is being used up on digestion. The blood supply to your brain is reduced because the stomach requires more blood for extra digestion.
- Overeating is a major cause of obesity and heart disease.

Why We Overeat

- Instinct tells us when we are hungry and, therefore, when to eat. It did 1000 years ago and it still does today. The body hasn't changed in the last 1000 years but something has changed—the quality of our food. Our food is grown in depleted soils and then this poor quality food is processed to further reduce the nutrient content. Finally, we heat it to kill off any nutrients which may be left. Your body knows when it's not getting sufficient nourishment and it maintains its appetite so you will keep eating until you are sufficiently nourished. Of course, this means eating a lot more than 1000 years ago. We need to eat twice as much to get the same amount of nutrients.
- Chemicals are often added to processed foods to stimulate our appetite artificially.
- Psychological problems, such as depression, can also lead to overeating.

How To Prevent Overeating

- Eat more natural foods, such as fruit, etc. The high nourishment value of these foods will satisfy the appetite centre in your brain more quickly than processed foods. Also, because you are eating less, your body will

digest the food more efficiently. Good digestion means your body is better nourished, and leads to a further reduction in appetite.
- Eat slowly. Again, this leads to more efficient digestion, improved nourishment and hence reduced appetite.
- Spread your food intake over several small meals rather than two or three big meals. For example, have small snacks of fruit in between your main meals. This also leads to better nourishment.
- Aerobic (fitness) exercise has been scientifically shown to reduce appetite.

HOW TO LOSE WEIGHT QUICKLY AND SAFELY

Eat fruit only for one day every week. Although fruit is low calorie, it is nutritious and bulky and therefore filling. This means you should not feel hungry.

Since fruit is also delicious, this is a very pleasant way of speeding up weight loss. Also, because it is only for one day a week, your body will not regard this as a familiar situation and so will not slow its metabolism down in order to preserve fat.

Another advantage of this one-day-a-week fruit regime is that it will start to eliminate toxins from your body. In other words, you will become healthier as well.

I suggest that you have watermelon or oranges for breakfast, since these fruits are very powerful toxin eliminators and you are taking advantage of the body being in its eliminative cycle at this time of the day. During the day eat whatever fruits you like or are in season. For the evening meal I suggest bananas because they produce a 'full' feeling which will help you get a good night's sleep! Since your body is accustomed to going to bed on a full stomach, your sleep may be disturbed if it is not full.

If you want to lose weight quickly you should also increase your exercise duration and frequency—at least until you have achieved your ideal slimming level. Once you have done this you can return to your normal exercise program to maintain your ideal level. So, to lose weight quickly I suggest you exercise six days a week, for at least twenty minutes a session until you have achieved your aim.

If you are over thirty years old, remember to do different exercises on alternate days. On three days a week do the double fat-burning exercises and on the other days you can do some purely aerobic exercise (walking, jogging, aerobics).

THE IDEAL NUTRITIONAL PROGRAM

The two basic principles of a good nutritional program, are to *keep it simple* and *avoid extreme diets*.

If you follow the general nutritional program below, there will be no need to worry about counting kilojoules, food combinations, or the correct amount and proportion of protein, carbohydrates and fat.

Breakfast

Fruit and wholegrain cereal. It's best to eat fruit immediately on arising, and then cereal about half an hour to one hour later. This allows the fruits to clean your system out before you eat the cereal. In addition, citrus fruits and cereal do not combine well and it's best to separate them.

Melons or oranges are excellent since they are powerful toxin eliminators as well as being a good source of natural sugar (fructose) for energy. Of course, you can always make a fruit salad; you can use some canned fruit but make most of it fresh fruit.

Lunch

Most people find sandwiches are convenient for lunch. They can be salad based or you may like to try banana sandwiches. Banana sandwiches increase your fruit intake and are very low in fat. They are an ideal combination because both bread and bananas are carbohydrates. There's also no need to butter the bread, since banana gives the bread a creamy texture flavour similar to butter. It's an ideal slimmer's meal and very nutritious.

Use wholemeal or multigrain bread rather than white bread. Vogel's wholemeal and sesame seed bread is great; it's 100 per cent wholemeal; stoneground flour is used (preserves the nutrients); and it contains nutritious sesame seeds.

Evening Meal

This is the best time to eat your protein and vegetables. Good protein sources are fish, meat, cheese, eggs, nuts, beans and soya bean products.

Don't eat an excessive amount of meat—fish is much better.

Vegetables should include salad because raw food is more nutritious than cooked food. Vegetables should be cooked by microwave, steaming or quick stir-frying. Boiling destroys most of the nutrients.

Snacks/Tea Breaks

Fruit is best!

Twenty Strategies to Prevent Overeating

1 Choose a photograph of yourself in which you look particularly fat and put it in a prominent place in the kitchen.

2 Stay as relaxed as you can; remember, in moments of stress you are likely to want to eat.

3 Buy one outfit in a size smaller before you start your diet.

4 Keep your fridge stocked with carrot, cucumber and celery to cope with those hunger pangs.

5 Do not cut out meals; cut down on quantity instead.

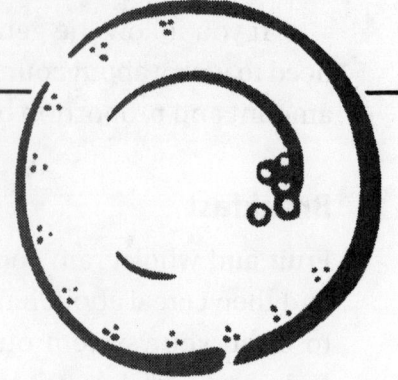

6 Leave a little food on your plate.

7 Before dining out, decide what you are going to eat. Don't read the menu.

8 Never eat fried food.

9 Flavour food with herbs and lemon juice. Avoid sugar, excess salt, alcohol and artificial flavourings.

10 Wrap food in foil for refrigeration so that you can't see it and therefore, hopefully, you won't be tempted by it.

11 Keep a chart of your measurements and fill it in once a week.

12 Don't shop for groceries on an empty stomach. Make a list and stick to it.

13 Never eat anything after dinner.

14 Eat desserts only on weekends—one way to limit problem foods without depriving yourself altogether.

15 Toss offending foods out of your kitchen and stock up on raw vegetables, fresh fruit, low-kilojoule dry biscuits, tomato juice, low-fat yoghurt and cottage cheese.

16 Learn to love water. Coffee and tea can give you caffeine jitters; ordinary soft drinks have sugar; diet drinks contain sodium.

17 When cooking, replace salt with spices and herbs.

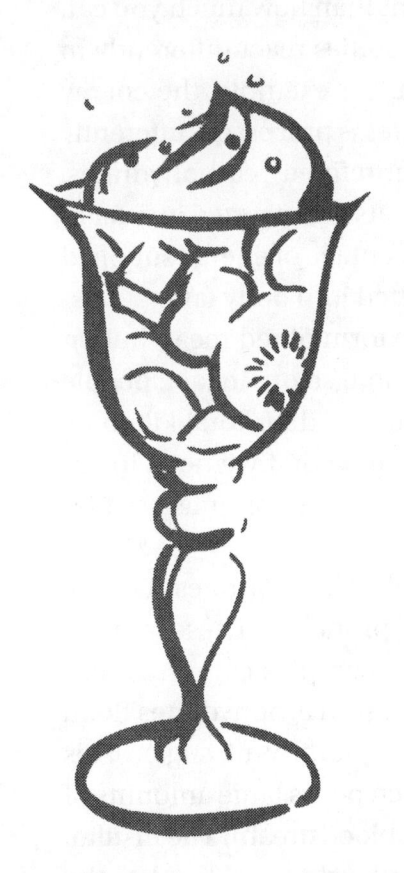

18 Cut out sugar. Use substitutes in coffee and tea; cook with cinnamon, nutmeg, lemon and fruit juices.

19 Reward yourself for your efforts—not just results—with something other than food.

20 Start exercising—now!

It's What and When You Eat That's Important

WHAT YOU EAT

Studies show that what you eat is more important than how much you eat. The type of food you eat may produce fat. Our bodies react differently to kilojoules supplied from different types of food. For example, the energy supplied by fats and simple (refined) carbohydrates is processed differently from the energy that comes from complex (unrefined) carbohydrates. Almost 100 per cent of the kilojoules supplied by fats is converted into fat to be stored in our body. Conversely, only a tiny percentage of energy supplied by complex carbohydrates and protein is converted into body fat.

Our diet is loaded with saturated fats in the form of red meat, butter, cheese, fried foods, cakes, biscuits, potato chips, and so on. In fact, people in Western nations derive between 40–50 per cent of their total kilojoule consumption from fats. Most nutrition experts agree that we need to cut this fat down to 20–30 per cent of total kilojoule intake to optimise our fat loss and then maintain our ideal weight.

The other main source of kilojoules is simple carbohydrates. That is, foods high in refined sugars and white flour products. These refined carbohydrates are metabolised differently to the complex carbohydrates supplied by wholegrains, fruit and vegetables. Simple carbohydrates flood the bloodstream with a sudden and excessive quantity of sugar. This triggers a dramatic response in the pancreas which pours large amounts of the hormone called insulin into the sugar-logged bloodstream. The insulin, which is responsible for controlling blood sugar levels, quickly takes the sugar from the blood into cells where it is converted into fat.

Complex carbohydrates, on the other hand, are digested slowly, releasing a gradual trickle of sugar into the bloodstream and producing a long-lasting energy boost. Most of this sugar remains available to be burned off through exercise and general bodily maintenance.

The complex carbohydrates of fruit, vegetables, and wholegrains aid your weight loss in other ways too. By supplying large amounts of bulky fibre, they quickly produce a full, satisfied feeling for longer after a meal.

WHEN YOU EAT

Kilojoules consumed in the first part of the day are burned up more efficiently than those consumed in the latter part of the day.

Studies carried out by American nutrition expert, Ronald Gatty, confirm this. In one experiment, one group of subjects took the bulk of their food in the mornings, while the other group took most of their food in the latter part of the day. Both groups ate whatever they wanted. The group eating late in the day gained about 0.25 kilograms per week. The early eaters actually lost weight at the rate of about 1.25 kilograms per week.

The main problem with eating late is that in the evening we tend to be sedentary—we are not burning up kilojoules by doing physical activity. Also, early in the day insulin levels are lower, and consequently less fat can be stored at this time and more kilojoules are made available to be burned during activity. Later in the day insulin levels are high and this makes fat storage easier. There are a number of other digestion-related hormones (such as adrenalin and glucagon) with similar time-related fluctuations which make digestion and energy use more efficient early in the day.

Simply eating the bulk of your total food intake before 1 p.m. is far more effective than dieting, and far better for your health. I suggest you eat your 'energy' foods such as fruit and wholegrains (bread/cereal) in the morning and at lunchtime, and eat low energy foods such as vegetables and protein for your evening meal.

Ten Foods to Help You Slim

The following foods are nutritious as well as being low in fat and high in fibre. The high fibre content creates a full feeling in your stomach so that you feel satisfied with less food. In addition, since these foods are highly nutritious, your body will require less food, and this will be reflected in a reduced appetite. Here they are:

Wholemeal Bread
Contrary to popular opinion, bread does not make you fat. Wholemeal bread is a great slimming food full of fibre and nutrients. Bread is only fattening when you add fattening things to it, such as butter, cheese or mayonnaise. Stick to toppings such as tuna, chicken, egg, fish fillets or salad.

Potatoes
Again, contrary to popular opinion, potatoes do not make you fat. Two or three potatoes will easily fill you up. Keep in mind too that when you feel full you will be less inclined to eat fattening processed or junk food. Obviously, your health will improve also.

Wholemeal Cereals
Like wholemeal bread, wholegrain cereals are high in fibre and nutrients and so give you that full, satisfied feeling. Cereals are even better than bread because the milk you add causes the fibre to swell inside your stomach, creating an even fuller feeling.

Examples of wholegrain cereals are 'Vitabrits', 'Weet-Bix', 'Weeties', raw muesli and oatmeal.

Fruit Milkshakes
These can be banana or avocado based. Fruit is a slimming food and again the milk causes the fibre in fruit to swell producing the fullness feeling. I suggest you use either soya milk or low-fat milk. If you use ripe bananas you won't need to add any sweetener, since the drink will be sweet enough.

Just place one glass of milk in a blender with one or two ripe bananas. If you like it cold, add a couple of ice-cubes.

As well as being a slimmer's drink, it's also nutritious and delicious.

Popcorn

It's best to use a hot-air popcorn-maker rather than one which requires oil. Popcorn is a good low-fat snack. It's also a favourite with the kids. It is preferable not to add sugar but a little salt for flavour is all right.

Fish

Fish has much less fat than meat and the fat it does contain, the omega-3 fats, are actually good for you. Studies show they actually lower your blood cholesterol levels.

You can buy delicious packeted, crumbed fish in the freezer section of supermarkets. All you need do is grill or oven cook it. There is no need to add extra oil because the fish will probably already have mono-saturated vegetable oil added, usually canola oil. Try making fish-burgers. Just fill a wholemeal bun with crumbed fish and lettuce and tomato. Put some mayonnaise on top of the fish—you can buy soya mayonnaise from health shops if you want to avoid cow's milk products.

Fruits

As already mentioned, fruit is an ideal slimmer's food: its fat content is non-existent and its bulk and high nutritional content satisfy your appetite.

Vegetables

For the same reasons as fruit, vegetables are also a slimmer's food.

Chilli

Chilli assists slimming by increasing the body's metabolic rate. Just by adding a little chilli to your food you can burn up to 300 kilojoules. This is referred to as 'a diet-induced thermic effect'. In addition, it's been my observation that people who start to use chilli, start to lose their craving for sweet food. They develop a taste for hot, spicy foods instead of sweet foods.

You can add chilli to most of your dishes; it goes especially well with stir fried dishes and other Chinese dishes. As a bonus, chilli is also rich in vitamins, minerals and enzymes, stimulates the circulation, and assists digestion by stimulating the production of hydrochloric acid in the stomach.

Mineral Water and Herbal Teas

I suggest you use these drinks to replace at least part of your alcohol consumption. Alcohol is rich in dead calories; it makes you fat without providing any nourishment. Even drinking coffee would be preferable to drinking alcohol—go easy with the sugar though.

Tips for Losing Fat Quickly and Keeping it Off

INCIDENTAL EXERCISE ASSISTS SLIMMING

Incidental exercise refers to small amounts of exercise carried out as part of day-to-day functions such as walking to the bus or train station.

The extent to which this helps depends on the amount of incidental exercise carried out. The more you do, the more fat you lose.

EXERCISE BEFORE A MAIN MEAL

If you increase your large-muscle activity (aerobic exercise), the level of your blood glucose will rise as glucose production in the liver increases to compensate for muscle glycogen depletion. This rise in blood glucose causes a reduction in appetite. In theory, this means you will eat less if you exercise just before your main meal.

WATER RETENTION IN WOMEN

The retention of water occurs chiefly because of hormonal changes during a woman's menstrual cycle. This could mean a temporary weight gain of up to about two kilograms, usually a few days before a menstrual period.

If you change your lifestyle to include good nutrition and exercise, along the lines described in this book, this problem should disappear. If it persists, your doctor may prescribe a mild diuretic to help eliminate the fluid.

You should not take water-reducing tablets; if they seem to make you lose weight, it is only because they interfere with your normal bodily functions.

Be careful to avoid accumulating extra water when there is no need. For example, both excess salt and alcohol lead to extra water retention.

ARE YOU DRINKING ENOUGH WATER?

Next to air, water is the element most necessary for survival. A normal adult is 60–70 per cent water. We can go without food for almost two months, but without water for only a few days. Many people do not drink sufficient water, and therefore live in a dehydrated state.

If you don't drink sufficient water, your body won't break down fat adequately. In addition, your body will try to conserve water and this causes water-retention problems.

You need to drink about six 240 millilitre glasses a day. If you eat a lot of fruit, you are getting the purest and best mineral water there is, and you'll only need to drink about two glasses of water a day. If you exercise, you'll need to drink an extra glass of water before you exercise to replace fluid lost from perspiration.

THE NATURAL NUTRIENT AND FOOD WHICH REDUCES YOUR APPETITE

A new study indicates that drinks sweetened with fructose—the kind of sugar found in fruit and fruit juices—curbs the appetite.

Judith Rodin of Yale University compared the hunger-curbing effects of plain water with three lemonade-flavoured drinks containing different sweeteners on 24 men and women. The drinks were consumed 40 minutes before a buffet-style lunch.

Drinks flavoured with glucose (which is found in table sugar) caused a slightly increased kilojoule consumption compared with people who drank plain water. Fructose-sweetened drinks, however, caused the subjects to eat 10–15 per cent fewer kilojoules after consuming the fructose. In addition, the subjects tended to pick fewer high-fat foods after a fructose drink.

Obviously the fruit sugar, fructose, has a satisfying effect on the appetite. You can buy fructose from health shops. My suggestion is to eat a piece of fruit about half to one hour before lunch and the evening meal.

This way you are getting good nourishment, as well as reducing your appetite.

SPECIFIC VITAMINS THAT HELP REDUCE FAT

Vitamin B$_5$
Fat is burned up at a much slower rate if vitamin B$_5$ is in short supply.

Vitamin B$_6$
This is required by the body to convert stored fats into energy.

Vitamin E
Adequate levels of vitamin E ensure that fats are burned at twice the normal rate.

Phosphatidyl Choline
This substance stimulates fat burning. Good sources are: lecithin, raw egg yolk and soya beans.

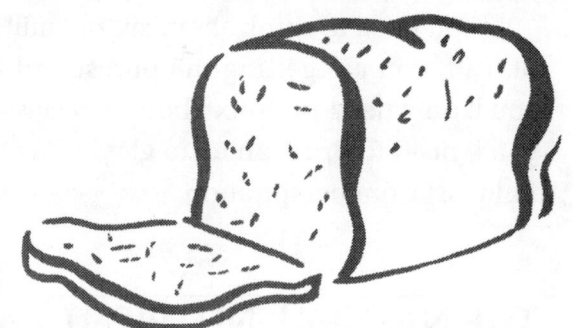

IS BREAD FATTENING?

The answer is: it depends. If you eat bread with the usual spreads such as butter and margarine, and have cheese or jams for example, then yes it is fattening. But bread on its own is not fattening.

To give you some idea how relatively low in fat bread is, just consider that it would take fifteen slices of bread to equal the kilojoules in one T-bone steak.

Olaf Michelson, a professor of blood science and human nutrition, demonstrated that bread can actually help control weight. Overweight young men were told to consume twelve slices of bread a day in addition to whatever else they ate. They were also advised to avoid high-kilojoule foods. The bread made them too full to desire these foods anyway. After eight weeks, the men who ate ordinary white bread had lost an average of 6.2 kilograms, while those who ate high-fibre bread had lost an average of 8.8 kilograms.

So eat plenty of bread—preferably wholemeal bread, since it's very nourishing—but avoid the spreads.

ARE POTATOES FATTENING?

The answer is no. In fact, the fat content in 2.5 kilograms of potatoes equals the fat content in just ten roasted peanuts.

As with bread, it's a common misconception that potatoes are fattening. They are only fattening when you add high fat foods, such as sour cream or cheese, or cook them with fat as in roast potatoes or french fries. You can add low-fat yoghurt and chopped chives, since this is adding only about 42 kilojoules.

Potatoes are actually a very nourishing low-fat food, so eat plenty of them. The healthiest way to cook them is to bake them in an oven, or even better, cook them in a microwave where they only take a few minutes.

LOSING WEIGHT AND IRON

Studies by the American College of Sports Medicine have shown that it is harder to lose weight if you are iron-deficient. This is significant since 10–15 per cent of Australian women are iron-deficient. Anemia caused by iron deficiency is one of the commonest deficiency disorders in women but rarely occurs in men. This is because women lose blood with menstruation during the reproductive years of their lives.

You may be lacking iron if you become pale and feel tired; blood tests will confirm anemia. Iron cannot be produced in the body therefore it is essential to eat some foods that contain iron.

The best sources of iron are dried peas and beans, wholemeal flour, green vegetables and meat.

BUTTER OR MARGARINE—WHICH IS BEST?

Butter

Butter's main drawback is that it contains mostly saturated fat (the bad fat), and cholesterol. It contains only a very small amount of essential fatty acids, and so has no nutritional value except to provide energy. It also concentrates pesticides five to ten times more than margarine.

On the positive side, butter is relatively stable when it is exposed to light, heat and oxygen compared with vegetable oils (margarine). It's also easily digested and pleasant to taste.

Margarine

Although margarine is advertised as high in essential polyunsaturated oils, these oils have been changed in the manufacturing process. These altered oils are harmful. There is evidence that these oils may be involved in cardiovascular disease and cancer.

To make matters worse, margarine may contain a number of additives, such as colouring, emulsifiers and flavourings including MSG.

So, which is best? In terms of trying to slim, butter and margarine are as bad as each other, since they are both 100 per cent fat. In terms of health, they are also bad news. Both lack decent amounts of essential fatty acids and both have a fairly high cholesterol content.

My choice would be to use butter in strict moderation. This choice is based on the fact that butter is a partly natural product, and is better tasting and more digestible. Margarine has only two advantages: it's cheaper; and spreads better.

HEALTHY SNACKS

Don't be frightened of snacking. Studies have shown that if you snack on the right foods, you will actually lose fat. This is due to your metabolic rate being maintained at a higher level throughout the whole day, and the fact that you will eat less at your main meals.

Examples of good healthy snacks are: fruit (not dried fruit or fruit juice), homemade banana milkshakes made with skim milk or soya milk (no sugar added), wholemeal fruit buns, raw nuts and popcorn made at home with a hot-air popcorn-maker.

DON'T SKIMP ON LUNCH

Reducing food intake at lunch is an approach adopted by many people as a means of weight control. However, research on reduced lunch size, whether in terms of carbohydrates or fat, has shown that the body tends to compensate over the rest of the day. You may not realise it but you consume more food at other times to reach the same total daily energy input.

One study, carried out at Johns Hopkins University, varied fat and carbohydrate intake in a small group of live-in subjects over thirteen days. While reduced meals tended to decrease the energy input, there was an unconscious compensation for this later in the day when subjects were allowed free access to food.

On a positive note, it was found that when the lunch was lower in fat, subjects compensated by eating more carbohydrates during the rest of the day. This is beneficial, even though the energy intake was the same, since excess fat is detrimental to health.

EVENING MEAL—EAT A SALAD FIRST

Salad is very low in calories and being very high in nutrition and fibre, it will soon fill you up. If you eat other food first, you will tend to fill yourself up on the tastier food, and probably be too full to eat a salad. You are then missing out on good nourishment and a good 'slimming food'.

Salad—What To Be Wary Of

Salads are very low in fat and very nutritious but, of course, you have to watch what is added to the salad. Avoid mayonnaise and salad dressings. Coleslaw and potato salad usually have a lot of high-fat dressings.

If you must flavour with a dressing, choose a low-kilojoule one. Remember that one tablespoon of ordinary salad dressing or mayonnaise is around 670 kilojoules.

SHOPPING FOR LOW-FAT FOODS

Skim milk—has 200 less kilojoules per cup than whole milk.
Tuna—a medium size can of tuna packed in water has about half the kilojoules of one packed in oil.
Sour cream—substituting plain yoghurt for sour cream saves more than 1200 kilojoules per cup.
Margarine—diet-brand margarines contain half the fat of standard margarines.

ALCOHOL

It's best to drink alcohol in strict moderation. The sugar in alcohol is converted to a type of fat called triglycerides. This is then stored in the body's fat reserves.

A NATURAL LOW-ENERGY SWEETENER

Aspartame, which is the scientific name for 'Nutrasweet' and 'Equal', has been around for some time. It contains no kilojoules. Together with saccharin it seems to provide a low-energy substitute for people with a sweet tooth. A major advantage of aspartame which is now being appreciated by nutritionists is that it happens to be an amino acid (a naturally-occurring unit of protein) with strong sweet properties.

As a natural product, aspartame has more market appeal and possibly the market edge over the other low-energy sweeteners. The downside is that, unlike saccharin, aspartame is not resilient in cooking. These sweeteners have been given a clean bill of health from most food and nutritional authorities if they are taken in moderation.

VARY YOUR DISHES

Dietary-induced thermogenesis is the term given to energy used up (and given off as heat) following the digestion of food. It forms a significant part of daily energy use (around 15–20 per cent) and any increase in thermogenesis may increase your fat loss.

European research with a group of women compared the effects of different types of food on thermogenesis. It was found that thermogenesis was higher with unfamiliar food, that is more kilojoules were burnt up in digesting unfamiliar food. The message is to vary your dishes.

Fifty Painless Ways To Cut Kilojoules

1 Top your baked potato with a tablespoon or two of low-fat yoghurt and finely chopped onion or chives. At little more than 42 kilojoules this topping saves about 170 kilojoules on even the smallest (7 gram) knob of butter.

2 Mix soda water—half and half—with your orange juice. More refreshing! Remember, even 150 millilitres of neat unsweetened juice costs you 191 kilojoules, so this is a worthwhile little saving.

3 Always wait for toast to cool before buttering. This way the bread absorbs less spread.

4 Instead of frying those frozen battered foods (cod and haddock fillets, chicken or fish fingers in batter, etc.) bake them without fat in a moderately hot oven 190° celsius. They taste just as crisp and good.

5 Quickly cool casseroles after cooking to lift off high-kilojoule fat. Or skim off fat with a metal spoon while casserole is still hot, removing the last traces with a piece of lightly applied kitchen paper.

6 Use matured cheddar cheese rather than a mild cheese for cooking.

7 Quench your thirst with water first, before turning to any kilojoule-supplying drink, and you will drink fewer kilojoules.

8 After browning mince in a frying pan, melt and drain off that high-kilojoule fat.

9 Make tea in the good old traditional teapot rather than by putting a teabag in your cup. This way you can enjoy at least two cups of tea with only one dash of milk! Most people use about 30 millilitres (84 kilojoules) in each cup of tea.

10 If you must make pies, roll the pastry as thinly as possible and only put pastry on top of the pie.

11 Always remove the skin after you have cooked chicken. A 250 gram joint is reduced from 763 kilojoules to 636 kilojoules when it is skinned. An average drumstick is reduced from 382 kilojoules to 340 kilojoules when the skin is removed.

12 For a very low-kilojoule cauliflower cheese, try this simple recipe. Just spread some boiled cauliflower with cottage cheese, season it and grill for a few minutes. You can have a big plateful for fewer than 425 kilojoules. Sprinkle a little paprika on top for colour and flavour.

13 You can use only three (not four) tablespoons of dried skimmed milk to make 600 millilitres and you will find this perfectly acceptable to put on your cereal. This gives you the lowest kilojoule milk of all at only 573 kilojoules per 600 millilitres compared to 848 kilojoules for ordinary skimmed milk.

14 If your family object to skimmed milk, try the 'sneaky' tactic of slimmers and water down the milk you serve in the jug. They swear (don't tell them) their families don't even notice when they add 150 millilitres of water to 450 millilitres of milk. This reduces 600 millilitres of milk from 1610 kilojoules to 1074 kilojoules.

15 Keep butter and margarine soft so that you spread far less. And always butter Ryvita crispbreads on the flat side so that you don't fill up the holes with extra kilojoules.

16 Make your own coleslaw by shredding 60 grams white cabbage, 30 grams grated carrot, one teaspoon finely chopped onion and mixing with a low-kilojoule coleslaw dressing and low-fat yoghurt. This costs just over 255 kilojoules compared with a carton of bought coleslaw in mayonnaise which costs from 742 kilojoules upwards.

17 Carefully drain all oil from canned fish. Either blot up any excess oil with kitchen paper or rinse the fish under cold water. If you like sardines canned in tomato just as much as those canned in oil, always choose the former. Sardines soak up some of the oil and are higher in kilojoules even when drained.

18 Use eating apples for making stewed apple, apple fool, apple sauce, etc. You can add much less sugar than with tart-tasting cooking apples, and you may find you don't need to sweeten at all. Tart-tasting fruits always encourage lavish use of sugar, and each extra 30 grams adds 475 kilojoules.

19 When using chicken joints in casseroles, skin them before cooking so that no fat is added to the gravy.

20 Grill all these items without any fat, they don't need it: sausages, fish fingers, bacon, beefburgers, rissoles, steak, chops and oily fish. Grill on a wire rack.

21 Spread sandwiches with cheese spreads or meat or fish pastes, instead of butter or margarine. The pastes and spreads take the dryness from the bread at a considerably lower cost in kilojoules. Butter is 890 kilojoules per 30 grams as compared to around 340 kilojoules for cheese spread.

22 For pouring cream use half cream and half milk, light sour cream or low-fat evaporated milk. You can buy 'half and half' milk in some States, where it is called Smoothy.

23 Instead of whipping cream for piping and topping trifles, use chilled low-fat evaporated milk. Use it as soon as you have 'whipped' it.

24 Buy thin-sliced rather than thick or medium-sliced loaves. In terms of psychological eating satisfaction, a slice is a slice and you are unlikely to miss the extra thickness. The difference in kilojoules is considerable, 275 for a slim slice, 425 for a medium slice, 551 for a thick slice (all from sliced large loaves).

25 When eating bought sandwiches in cafes, remove the top slice and scrape off as much butter as possible. Ask for unbuttered sandwiches when eating out and you will find that most cafes are ready to oblige.

26 Always grate rather than slice cheese into sandwiches and crispbreads—salads, too. Makes a little seem like a great deal more!

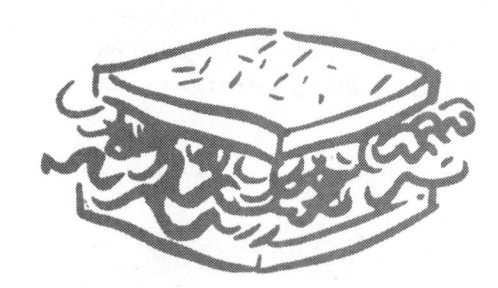

27 Try mixing one part low-kilojoule dressing to one part natural low-fat yoghurt. This is a perfectly painless way of serving an even lower-kilojoule salad dressing, 72 kilojoules compared with 106 kilojoules per tablespoon.

28 Try cottage cheese as a substitute for cream cheese. It has a similar creamy consistency and provides only 170 kilojoules per 30 grams compared to 530 kilojoules.

29 Enjoy the crusty crunch of a bread roll and tasty filling for only a few more kilojoules than the cost of the bread roll. Halve the roll and pinch out most of the soft bread before filling with a low-kilojoule food such as 60 grams of cottage cheese mixed with celery pieces, an egg scrambled with a chopped tomato and a pinch of mixed herbs (no butter), or 45 grams of canned salmon, drained and mixed with cucumber chunks.

30 When making fruit salads, use naturally sweet fruits like melons, eating apples, pears and grapes. You are far less likely to want to add sugar than if you use the 'sharp-tasting' fruits such as grapefruit and apricots.

31 Try using low-fat natural yoghurt instead of sour cream in goulashes and stroganoffs. A big kilojoule saving here.

32 Always thoroughly and crisply grill chops, sausages, beefburgers and bacon. Enormous kilojoule savings can be made by cooking off the maximum quantity of liquid fat.

33 When scrambling eggs, don't use butter or margarine—just add a tablespoon of milk for each egg.

34 When making moussaka or any other dish using sliced eggplants, don't fry them as instructed. Instead, blanch the sliced eggplant in boiling water for two to three minutes. An average 210 gram eggplant increases from 118 kilojoules to 1717 kilojoules when it is fried.

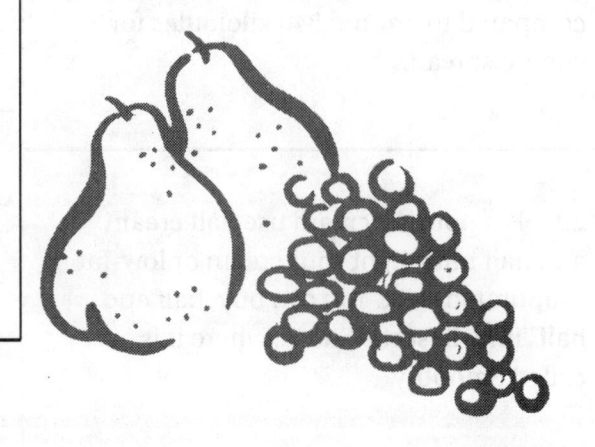

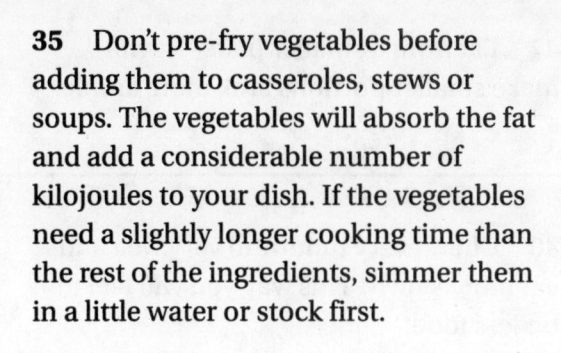

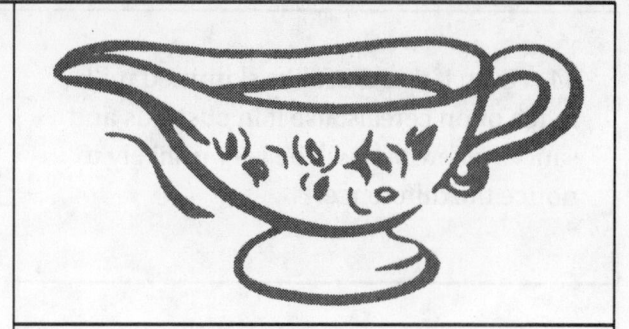

35 Don't pre-fry vegetables before adding them to casseroles, stews or soups. The vegetables will absorb the fat and add a considerable number of kilojoules to your dish. If the vegetables need a slightly longer cooking time than the rest of the ingredients, simmer them in a little water or stock first.

36 Make a policy of always using a little less fat than the recipe recommends when making sauces, casseroles and stews. Thirty grams less fat can save you 1081 kilojoules.

37 Make a policy of gradually getting to like dessert recipes a little less sweet. So always use a little less sugar than the recipe recommends in sauces, custards, mousses, stewed fruit recipes, and fruit pies. You can train yourself.

38 Try parmesan cheese, instead of ordinary cheeses, when you want to sprinkle cheese on a cooked dish or soup. Like matured cheddar, it has a strong flavour, so a little goes a long way.

39 Cut roast potatoes in big (rather than small) chunks before cooking so that they absorb fewer fatty kilojoules. The same 'big is better' rule applies to chips. Frozen crinkly-cut chips absorb most fat of all.

40 To make thick gravy, without fat, thicken stock by blending in cornflour and colour with a few drops of gravy browning. Saves a vast number of kilojoules on that traditional thick gravy made from blending flour into the roasting-pan juices and fat.

41 To make a very low-kilojoule fruit juice, purée seeded cubes of ripe watermelon, only 13 kilojoules per 30 grams, in your blender. You get 150 millilitres of watermelon juice for only 127 kilojoules.

42 Poach eggs in water in a shallow pan rather than using a poacher with compartments which have to be greased.

43 Make white and cheese sauces by thickening skimmed milk with cornflour, instead of the roux method of using flour and fat.

44 Even if you don't like skimmed milk in tea or on cereals, use it in custards and sauces where you will be very unlikely to notice the difference.

45 Make a fat-free sponge rather than a butter cake. This is a good recipe: Beat two eggs with half a cup of sugar until thick and creamy. Fold in three-quarters of a cup of sifted self-raising flour and a tablespoon of boiling water. Turn into a twenty centimetre sandwich tin. Bake for twenty to twenty-five minutes in a moderate oven, 180° celsius. Gives you one of the lowest kilojoule cakes you can eat.

46 If you must fry mushrooms and tomatoes, fry them whole or halved rather than sliced. Gives you a lower-kilojoule fry-up.

47 Eat from a smaller plate—it will make smaller portions look more ample.

48 Chew every mouthful very well and eat more slowly. This way you will feel full on less food.

49 Eat as much fresh food as possible; packaged foods contain hidden kilojoules.

50 Eat wholemeal grains (bread and breakfast cereals). This will fill you up more and therefore you will eat less.

Part Four

Looking Even Better

Trimming Your Thighs

The exercises in this chapter are optional. The most important aim you should have is to do the five double fat-burning exercises because they cause fat loss all over the body including the stomach, thighs and buttocks.

The objective of these exercises is to tone up the muscles in the thigh area to produce a more firm contoured appearance. Remember, spot reduction doesn't work—you can only lose fat from all over your body.

I suggest that you don't start these exercises until you have done the double fat-burning exercises for several months. These exercises won't achieve much until you have lost some fat; they are, if you like, the fine-tuners.

Exercise 1

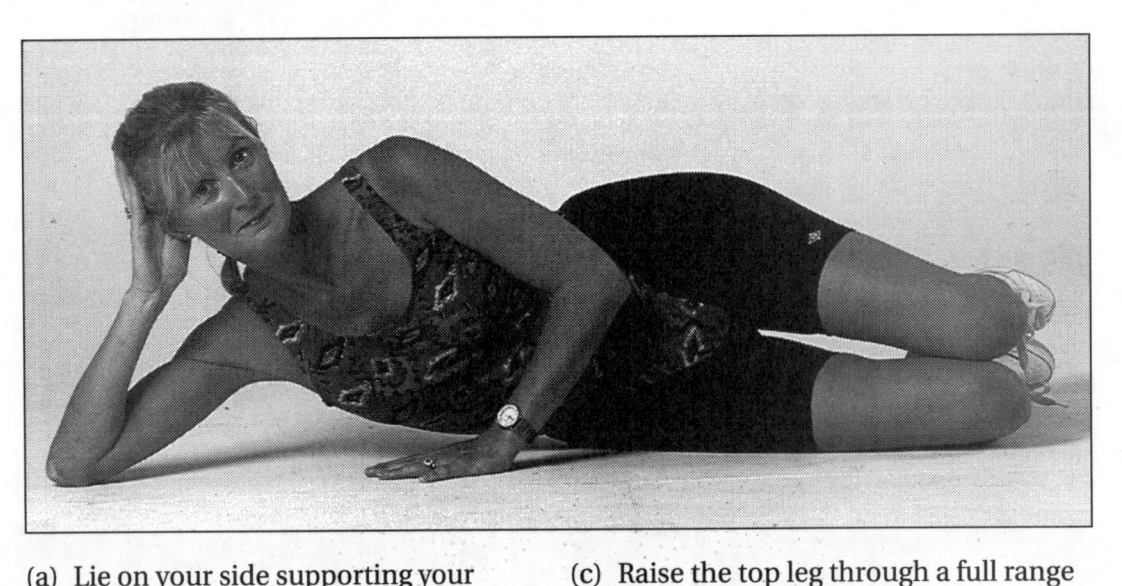

(a) Lie on your side supporting your head in your hand.

(b) Have both knees bent at a 45° angle to your hips.

(c) Raise the top leg through a full range without turning the hip.

Exercise 2

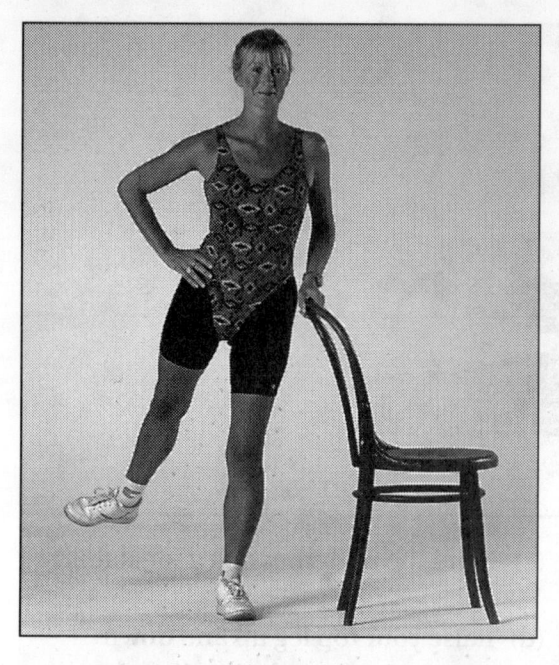

(a) To strengthen and trim your thighs, stand sideways-on to a support. Lift your outside hip and heel so that you feel a pull up in your waist.

(b) Lift your outside leg up to the side and rotate it inwards from the hip socket so that the knee is facing to the front. Draw your toes up towards you so that your foot is flexed. Now lift your leg up to the side so that you feel the outside of your thigh lifting your leg and squeezing round your hip socket. Lift sixteen times and then lift your leg to the side and swing it across in front of the leg you are standing on, then sweep it out to the side again. Repeat eight times.

(c) Turn back to the original position and lift your outside hip and heel.

(d) Slide your leg diagonally back, turn slightly out and lift sixteen times. Then sweep it forwards, following the diagonal line eight times. Repeat the sequence if you can, then face the other way and work your other leg.

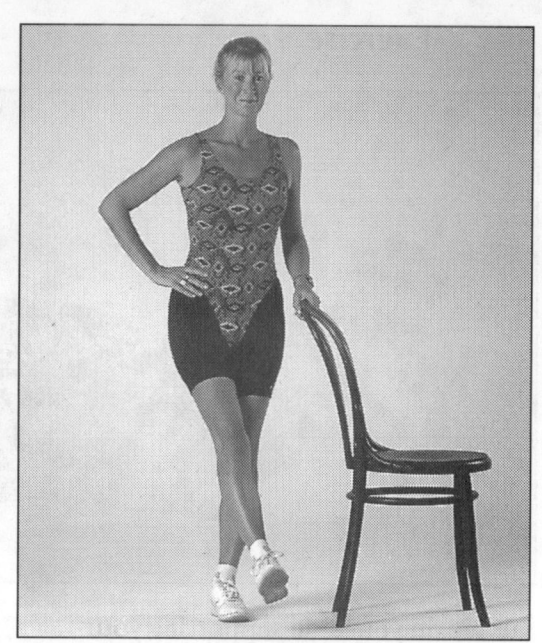

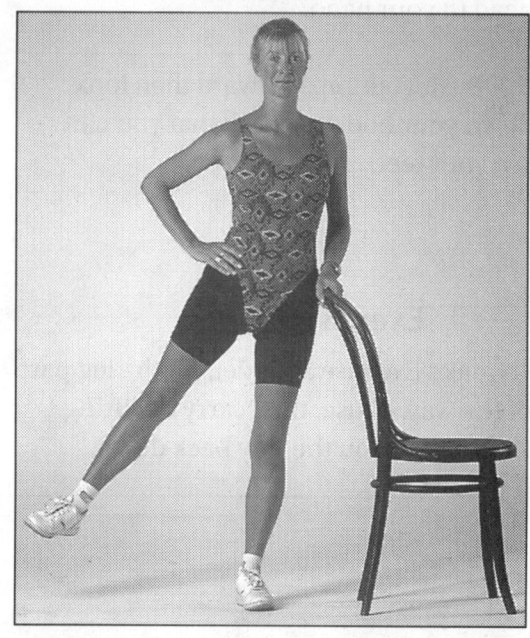

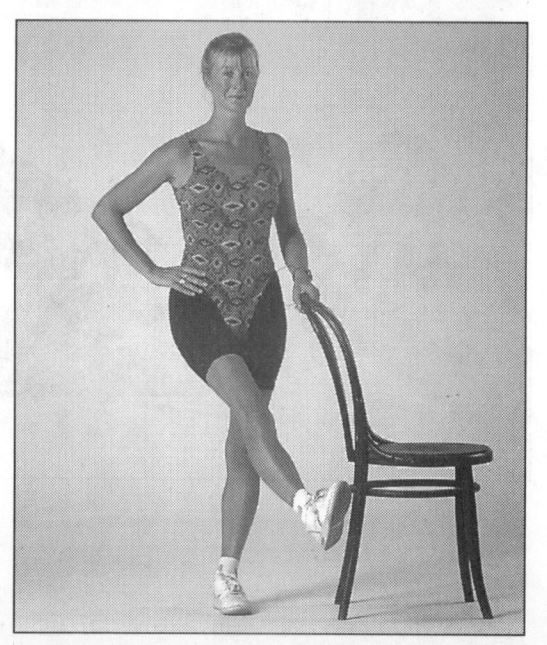

Exercise 3

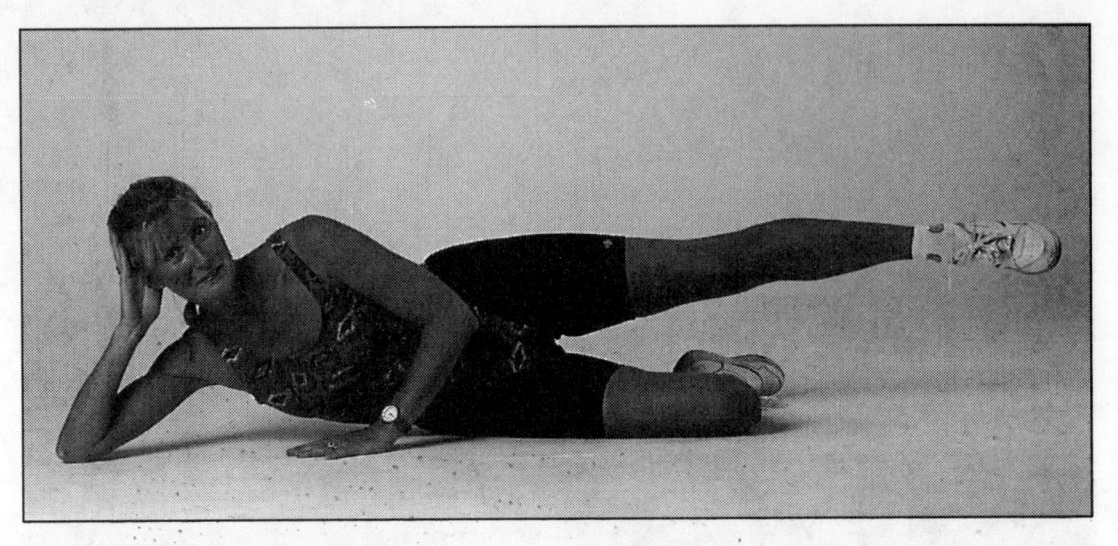

(a) Lie on your side supporting your head in your hand.

(b) Push your hips forward then look down your body to check that you can't see your feet.

(c) Bend the underneath leg for stability.

(d) Raise your top leg up and down keeping the kneecap facing directly forward.

Exercise 4

To make Exercise 3 harder, lift the leg part of the way, pause, then carry on lifting. Do the same on the way back down.

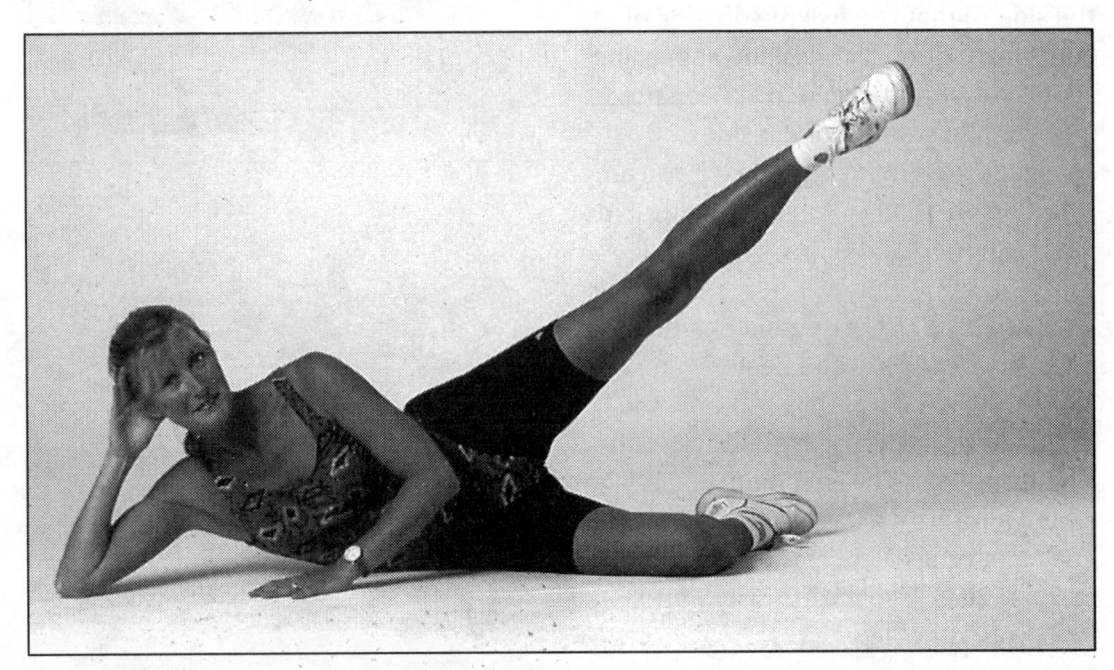

Exercise 5

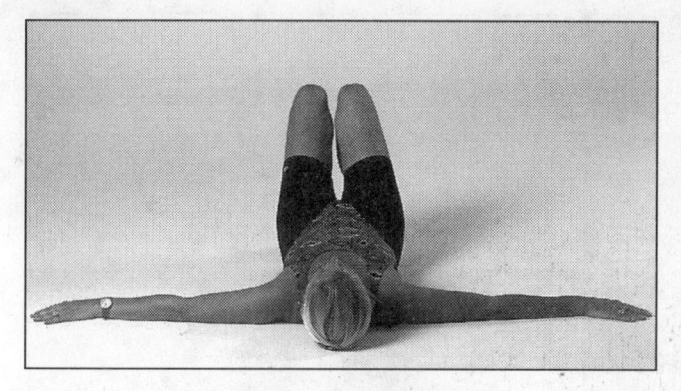

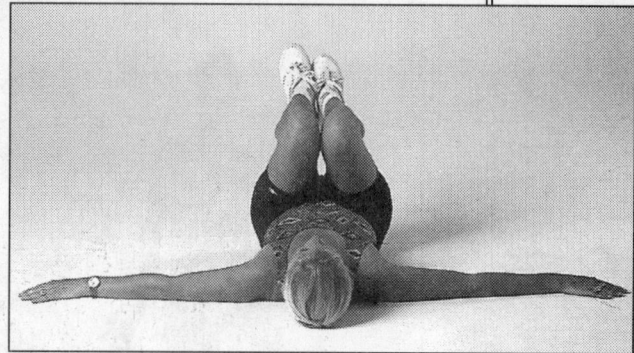

(a) Lie on your back on the floor with your arms out at the sides, palms down.

(b) Keeping your feet together, bring your knees up to your chest.

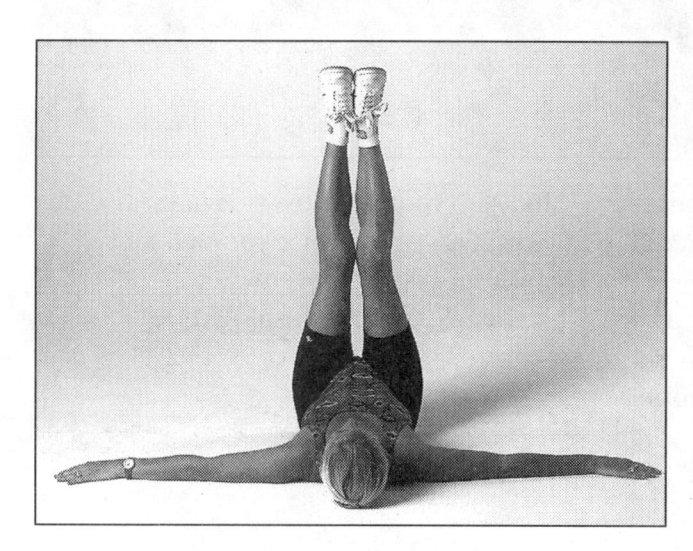

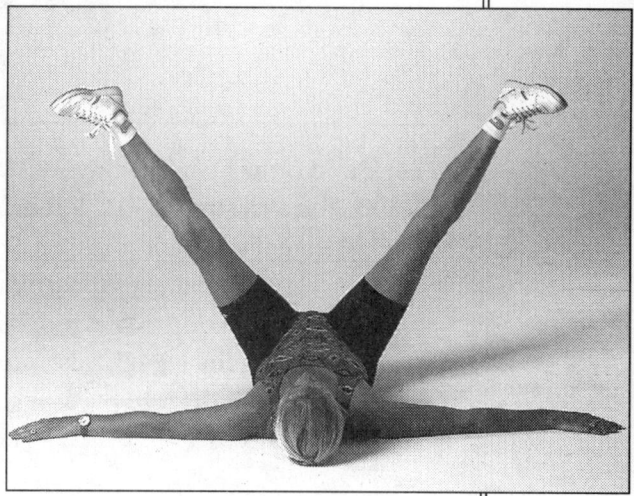

(c) Straighten your legs.

(d) With legs vertical, open them out sideways as far as possible, then close in a scissor action.

Repeat ten to fifteen times.

Exercise 6

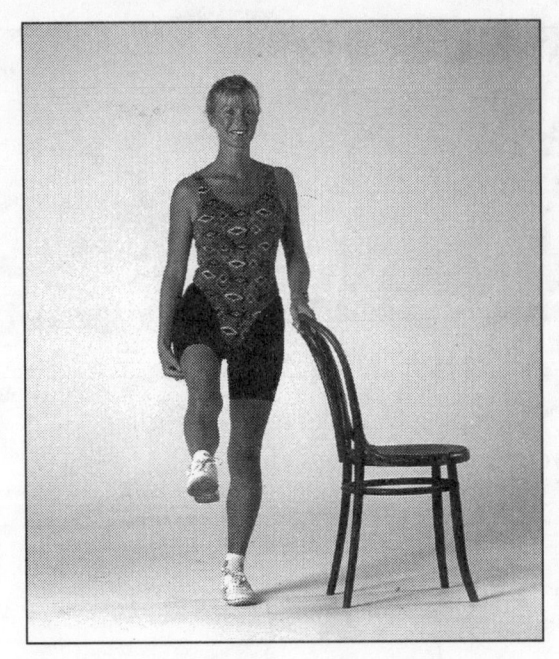

(a) Hold onto a chair with your right hand. You can stretch your left arm out for balance if you need. Pointing your toes, swing your left leg forward and backwards in a continuous movement. Then, keeping the leg up, take it around to the left side.

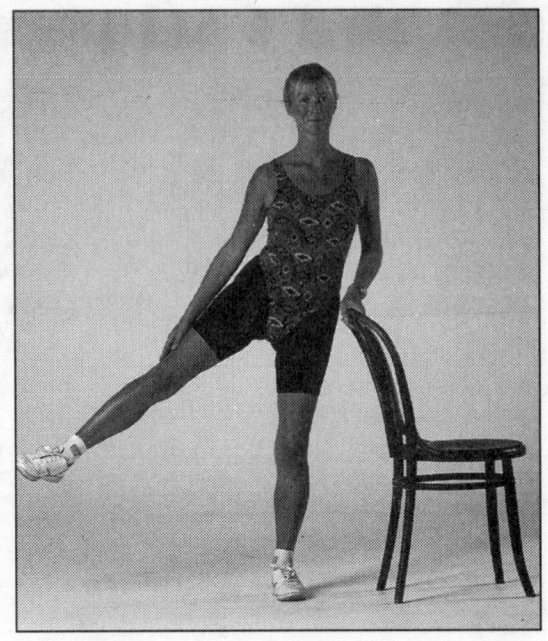

(b) With your leg lifted sideways, as shown, lower and raise your left foot in quick successive movements.

Repeat exercise with right leg.

Exercise 7

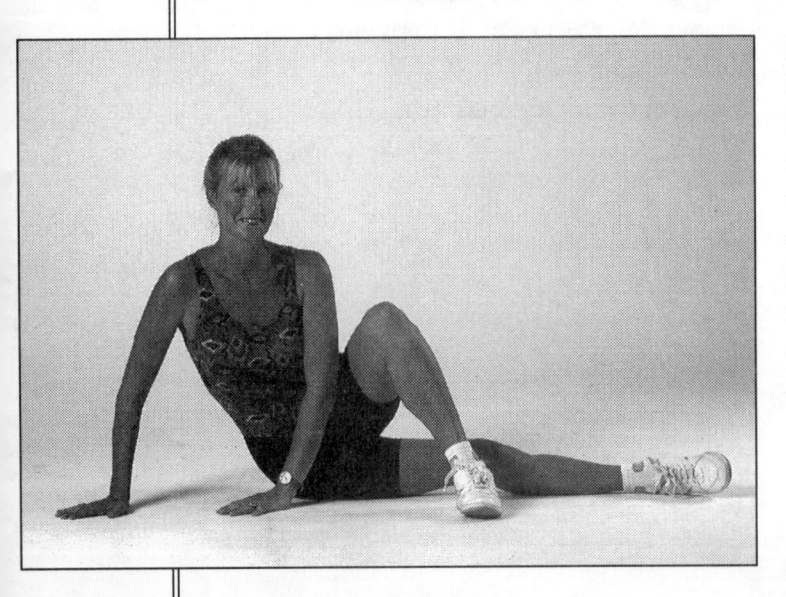

Sit on the floor, resting on your right buttock and right hand, with your right leg out straight, toes pointing down towards the floor and heel turned up towards the ceiling. Bend your left leg with toes pointing to the floor over your right knee. Hold tummy in and, flexing bottom muscles, slowly raise and lower your right leg as far as you comfortably can. Repeat five to ten times.

Repeat whole exercise with other leg.

Exercise 8

Sitting on the floor with legs slightly apart, stretch arms up. Bend forward, reaching as low as you comfortably can and stretch arms along your right leg towards the ankle. Return to a sitting position, then repeat movement towards left ankle. Continue for five repetitions.

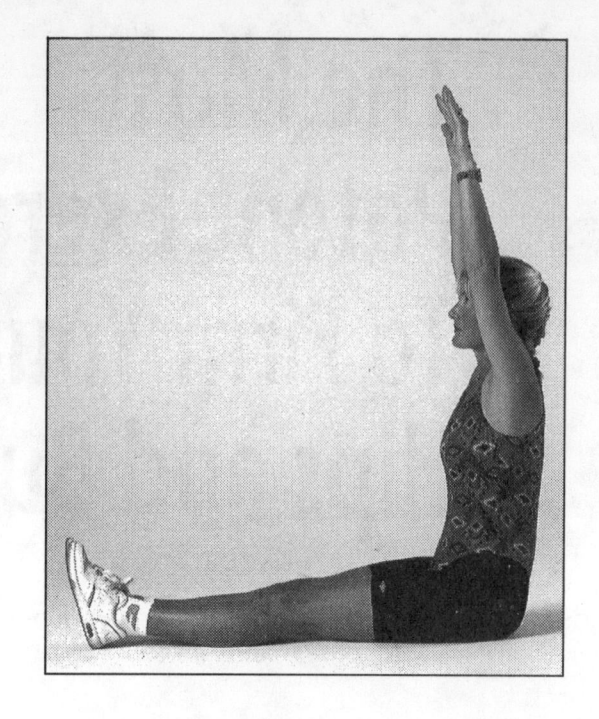

Trimming Your Thighs

The Most Potent Exercises To Firm Your Hips and Buttocks

Keep in mind the most important thing to do is the core set of the five double fat-burning exercises. If you do these five exercises you will then lose fat from wherever there are excess fat deposits—including the hips and buttocks.

The following exercises can be used to top up the double fat-burning exercises.

Exercise 1

If your work means that you have to sit a lot, you can do a simple exercise to counteract the tendency for the muscles of the buttocks to weaken and spread.

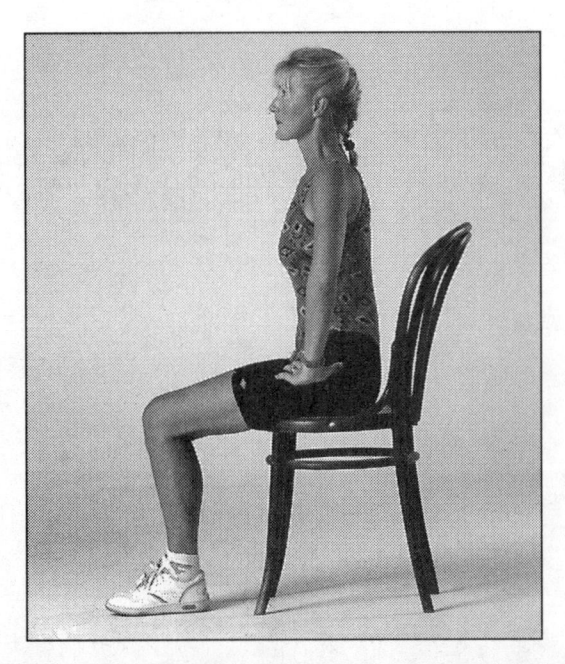

(a) First, sit upright with your feet flat on the floor. Press down into your feet so that your buttocks squeeze up underneath you. Squeeze and release for as long as you comfortably can, varying between quick and slow squeezes.

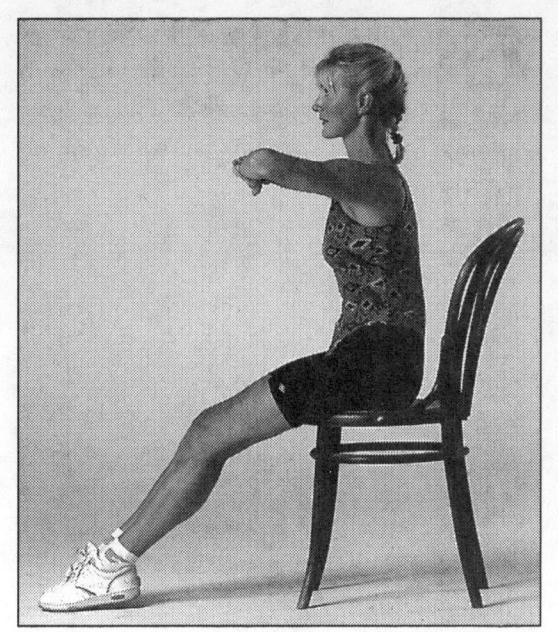

(b) From your upright position, tilt your pelvis back with your abdominal muscles held firmly in. Fold your arms in front of you, keeping your shoulders relaxed and downwards so that you are scooped out in the middle. Lift your feet a little way off the floor and squeeze your buttocks together underneath you. Stop if you feel any strain in your lower back.

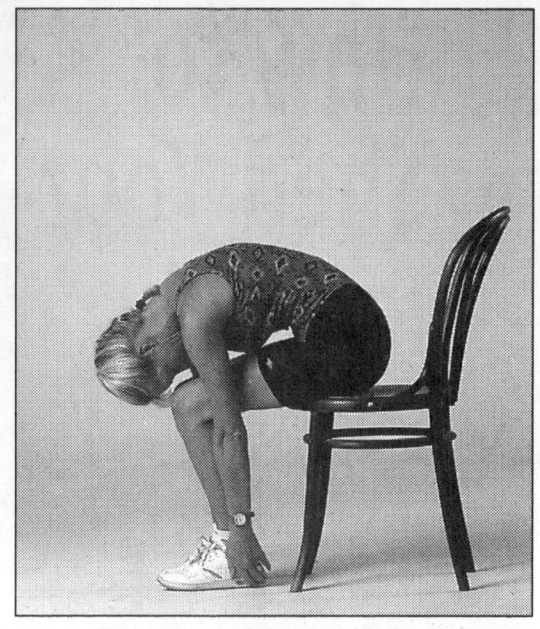

(c) Finally bend forwards from your hips, keeping your spine lengthened. With your chest resting on your thighs, drop your head down and take a deep relaxing breath. To come up, first lift your head so that it lines up with your spine and then come up straight with a flat back.

Exercise 2

Lie flat on your stomach, resting your chin on your hands. Lift one leg just off the floor, keeping hips facing the floor, and bend your leg. Keep your knee off the floor as you straighten the leg. Swap legs and repeat the sequence eight times.

Exercise 3

Kneel on the floor, resting on your elbows and knees. Pull in your stomach muscles. Extend one leg at a time and raise and lower it as slowly as you can. Change to the other leg after five repetitions.

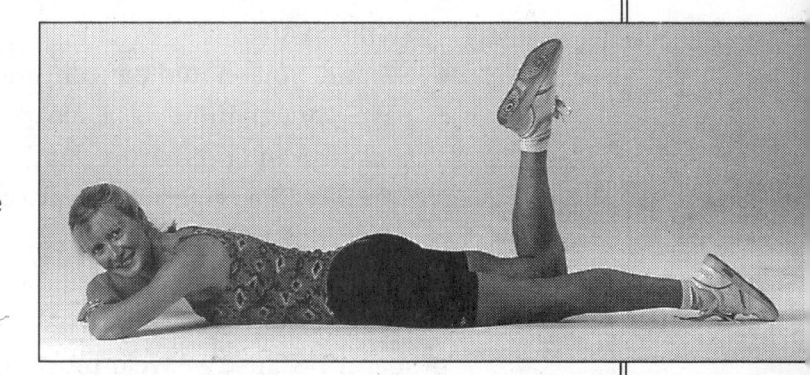

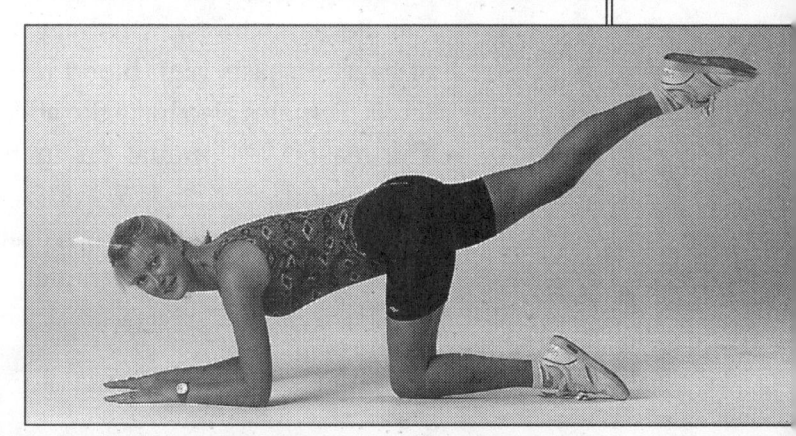

The Most Potent Exercises To Firm Your Hips and Buttocks

How to Shed Your Potbelly

WHY IT'S IMPORTANT TO REDUCE THE WAISTLINE

National Heart Foundation measurements of over 9000 Australians have shown that around 42 per cent of men and 24 per cent of women are carrying potentially dangerous abdominal fat (potbellies).

Special attention is given to the waistline for two reasons.

- First, in surveys people most often say they want to lose fat from their stomach area.
- Second, you should concentrate on your waistline because the studies have shown there is a close correlation between the size of your waistline and premature death.

In fact, the larger your waistline, the earlier you will die. Fat in other parts of the body does not have the same impact on your lifestyle. Insurance companies are well aware of this and partly assess your risk on the size of your waistline. The waistline is such an important indicator probably because we wear most of our fat in this area.

Research has shown that waistline fat in particular increases your risk of heart disease, high blood pressure and diabetes and high cholesterol levels. Females also have the added risk of cancer of the breast and uterus. The reason abdominal fat increases the risk of these diseases is not understood.

Research has also shown that individuals of both sexes tend to expand at the waist as they age although the tendency is more common in men.

THE CAUSES OF THE POTBELLY

In looking for causes of the potbelly, it was surprising to find that we are actually eating less than our grandparents did. What is different now is that the consumption of soft drinks, which are loaded with sugar, has increased over 100 per cent in the past decade. We are also less active physically; we walk less and use more labour-saving devices. The double fat-burning exercise program is the best way to compensate for our sedentary lifestyles.

So, while genetics and hormones do play a role, studies show that our lifestyle is the main factor in causing the bulging belly.

LITTLE KNOWN FACTS ABOUT THE POTBELLY

You Needn't Be Overweight To Have A Paunch

A person can be quite lean but still have too much abdominal fat relative to fat elsewhere.

There are two quick ways to tell whether you are too big around the middle.

- Stand up straight and lower your gaze to the floor; if you can't see your toes, you have a potbelly.
- A more scientific way is to calculate your waist-to-hip ratio. This is your minimum waist measurement (taken while standing) divided by your maximum hip measurement (taken around the buttocks). If the ratio exceeds 0.85 for women or 0.95 for men, it indicates abdominal obesity.

Women Get Potbellies Too

Protruding paunches tend to be associated with men because men generally deposit their fat in the abdominal cavity, while women typically gain in the hips and thighs. While this is true, both sexes can have either kind of fat distribution.

Like men, women tend to exercise less as they get older and assume other responsibilities. Pregnancies also cause an increase in abdominal fat. As the number of pregnancies increases, so does the proportion of abdominal fat. Why this happens is not yet known. Some women may be genetically predisposed to abdominal fat, and this may show up after they become pregnant. Or it may have something to do with breast-feeding; since lactation depletes fat stores, women who don't breast feed may develop more abdominal fat.

You Don't Have To Starve

However, to lose a potbelly you have to reduce your fat intake. This is because, compared with protein and carbohydrates, fat is energy dense. Protein and carbohydrates give you about seventeen kilojoules per gram, whereas fat gives you thirty-seven—more than double.

Research also shows that fat kilojoules are more fattening than protein and carbohydrate kilojoules. This means if you eat the same number of kilojoules of fat and carbohydrates, you'll gain more weight eating the fat. This occurs because dietary fat can enter the cells directly, while carbohydrates have to be converted into fat to be stored. This conversion takes energy and burns kilojoules.

Our average fat intake is about 40 per cent of our total kilojoule intake. Healthwise this is dangerously high, in addition to producing excess fat. We need to reduce our fat intake to about 20 per cent of total kilojoule intake. Your health would improve, you would look younger, live longer and certainly become slimmer.

You don't have to go on a crash diet to achieve the 20 per cent level. During the week just cut out the high-fat foods (fried foods, margarine, butter, cheese, cream) and reduce your meat intake. You will have to cut out the foods containing these items, such as cakes, biscuits, ice-cream and chocolate. Allow yourself to have your favourite food on the weekend. This way you are breaking the high fat habit, but still have something to look forward to at the end of the working week. This way you don't feel as though you are missing out on what you really like. The mental aspect of slimming is also important.

Forget Sit-ups for Losing Fat

Sit-ups will do nothing to reduce a paunch. In a 1984 study, subjects who averaged 185 sit-ups a day for twenty-seven days made no change in abdominal obesity. Spot reducing doesn't work. The only way you lose fat is by losing systemic fat; that is, fat from your whole system including even your arteries.

The only effective way to lose systemic fat is to reduce your fat/sugar intake and do aerobic exercise.

Sit-ups do have a place. They will tone up your abdominal muscles but, keep in mind, it's the fat underneath the muscle which is causing the paunch. Sit-ups will not affect the paunch itself.

Aerobic and Muscle-stimulating Exercise Program

This is the most effective way to eliminate fat including the fat around the abdomen. It's the most potent way to increase the body's metabolic rate, which is the main factor in burning up fat. If you need motivation to exercise, remember that the increase in body metabolism during exercise lasts twenty-four hours a day, so you are burning up fat even while you are sleeping.

In relation to abdominal fat, recent research suggests that aerobic exercise reduces fat first and fastest in the abdomen. The men in one intensive six-month program lost twenty per cent of their abdominal fat—almost twice the amount taken off arms and legs.

The best results of all are achieved by doing the aerobic-muscle-stimulating exercise program as described in Part 2, pages 40–72. Once you have lost your potbelly, exercising three or four days a week, rather than six days, will be sufficient.

Replace Some of Your High Fat/Sugar Foods With Complex Carbohydrate Foods

In a recent study of 124 women who each lost five to eight kilograms by cutting down on dietary fat and sugar, 64 per cent lost fat preferentially from their abdomen. Abdominal fat is easier to lose than fat on the buttocks and thighs, since the fat cells on the abdomen are larger and have the most potential for size reduction by shrinking.

Try to include as many fruits, vegetables and wholegrain products (bread/cereal) in your diet as possible.

Reduce Your Alcohol Intake

Alcohol, like sugar, is empty calories. It produces fat without giving you any nourishment; it seems there really is such a thing as a beer belly. In a study of 1628 men and women in the United States, those who drank more than two alcoholic drinks a day had the largest waist-to-hip ratio (W.H.R.) which is how doctors quantify potbellies. The drinkers had roughly twice as many large ratios as the non-drinkers.

Stop Smoking

In the same study, researchers at Stanford University School of Medicine and the University of California, San Diego detected a similar effect from smoking. There were twice as many fat abdomens among the smokers compared with non-smokers.

THE EIGHT MOST EFFECTIVE STOMACH MUSCLE-TONING EXERCISES

Exercise 1: Abdominal Crunch

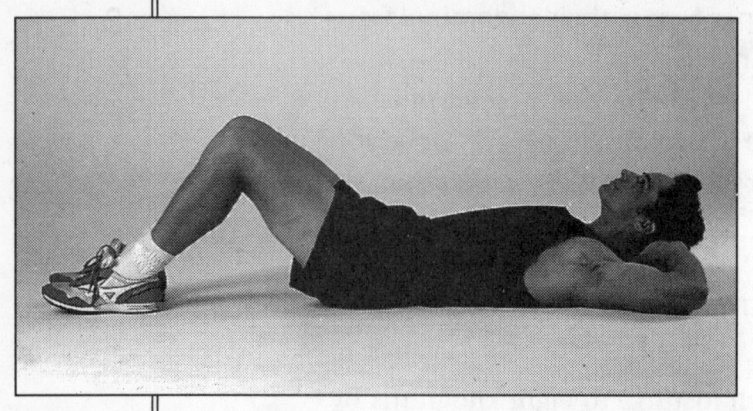

(a) Starting position: lie on your back, knees bent, feet hip-width apart and flat on floor. Interlock your fingers behind your head.

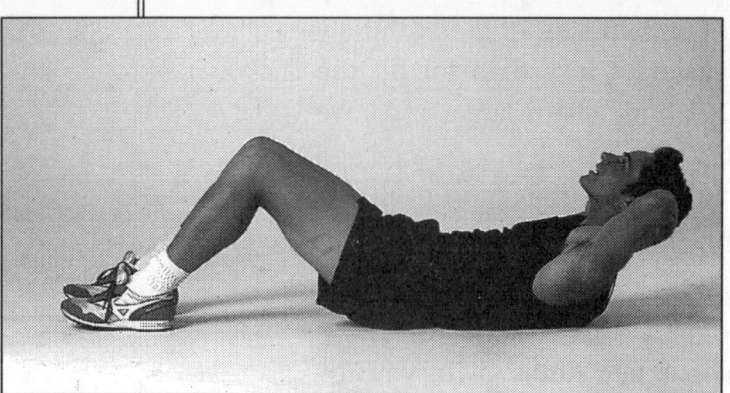

(b) Keeping your stomach muscles tucked in, lift your head and shoulders off the floor. Let your abdominal muscles pull you upward, not your neck and shoulders. Exhale during this step.

Inhale slowly as you return to the starting position.

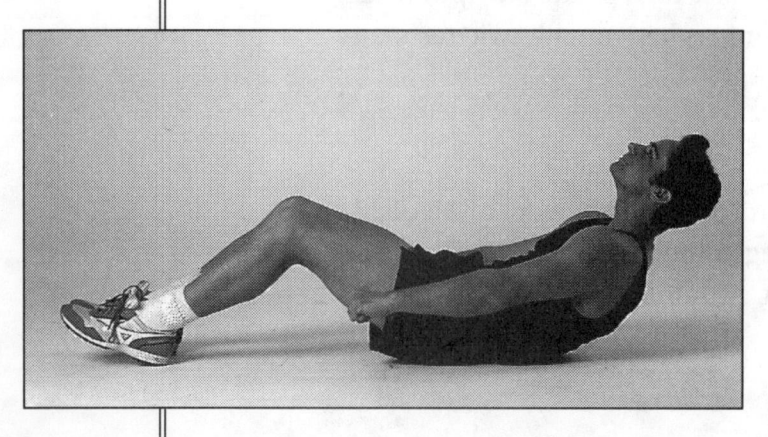

Exercise 2: Isometric Exercise

This exercise is the same as a sit-up, except you stop about half-way between sitting up and lying down and stay in that position for about eight seconds. Do this once, have a rest and repeat once more. Make sure you feel a strain on the stomach muscles.

If you find this too difficult at the start, do it without your hands behind your head. As your muscles get stronger, place your hands behind your head to hold yourself in a position closer to the floor.

Isometric exercises are the **fastest way** to build firm muscles.

Exercise 3: Isotonic Exercise

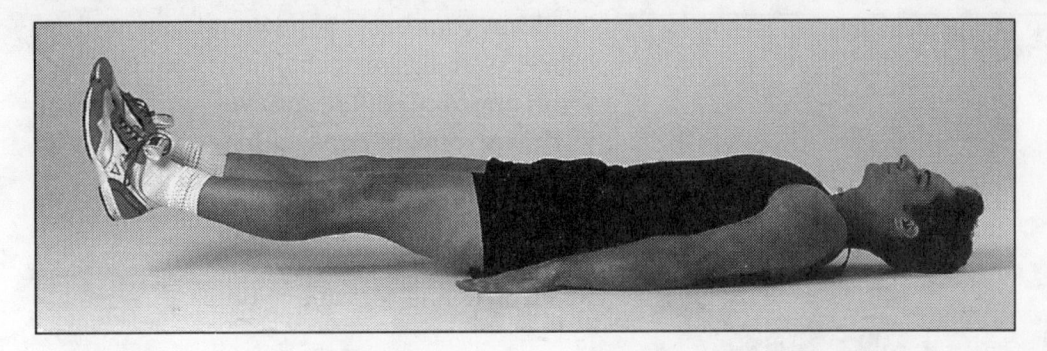

Lie on your back and lift both legs to about 45°, and then lower your legs to a count of about eight seconds. Repeat two more times.

While 'isometric' refers to building muscle while the body is in a stationary position, 'isotonic' refers to building muscle while the body is in movement. Both are extremely efficient methods for building firm muscle.

Exercise 4: Elbow-to-knee Touch

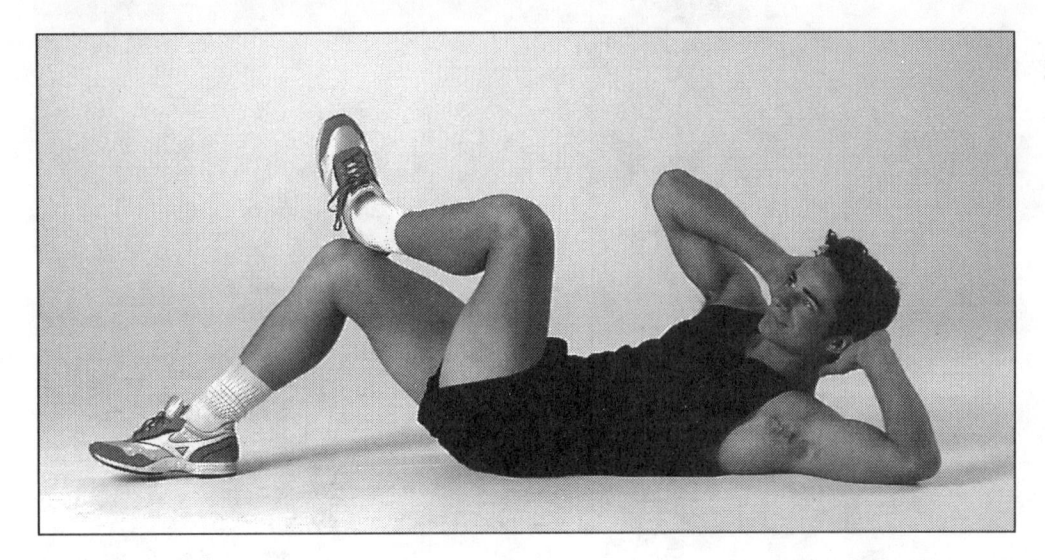

Lie on your back with your right knee bent and right foot flat on the floor. The left leg should be bent with your left foot crossed over your right knee. Interlock hands behind head.

Lift your upper body off the floor and reach for your left knee with your right elbow, keeping the left stationary. Exhale.

Inhale slowly as you return to the original position.

Exercise 5: Chair Exercise 1

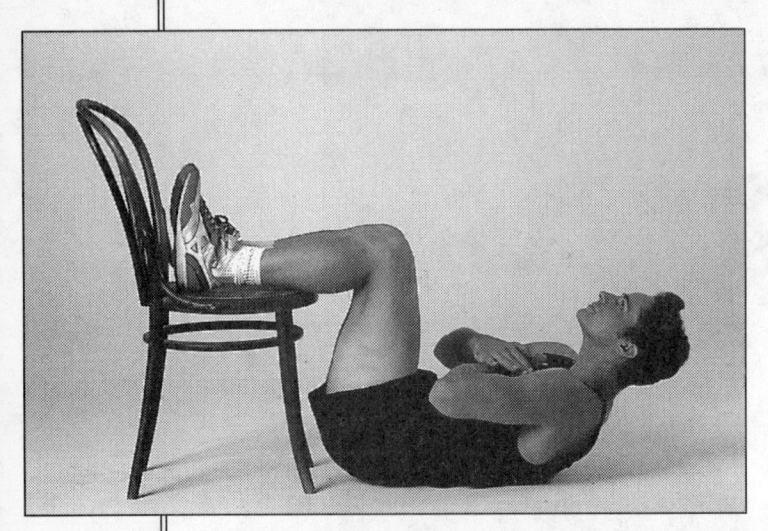

Lie on your back, bend your knees and rest your legs on a chair. Put your hands on opposite shoulders, eyes looking over the top of your head, chin level (not raised or flexed), raise your shoulders one-quarter of the distance between your knees and the floor. Hold for only three seconds and repeat five times.

Exercise 6: Chair Exercise 2

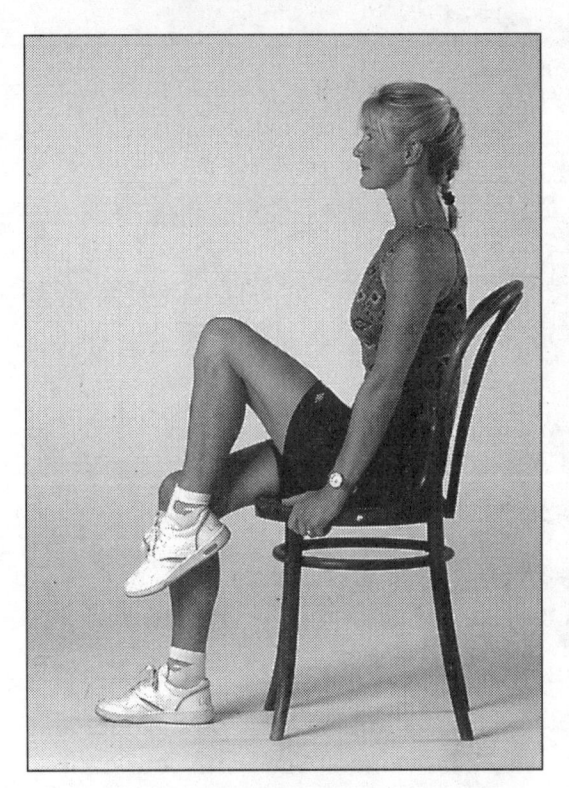

(a) To strengthen your abdominal muscles, start with your hands holding lightly to the sides of your chair. Lift first your right knee to your chest, lower it, and then lift your left knee. Repeat slowly and smoothly four times with each leg.

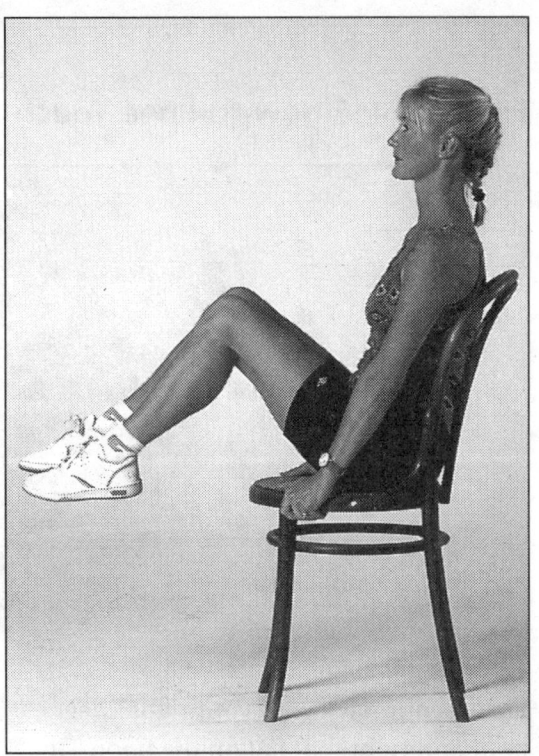

(b) When you feel comfortable with the previous exercise, try lifting both legs together in the same way, breathing out as you do so. Make sure you keep your hips tilted back and that your abdominal muscles are pulled in at the same time.

Exercise 7: Bike Ride

(a) Starting position: lie on your back, body weight supported on forearms.

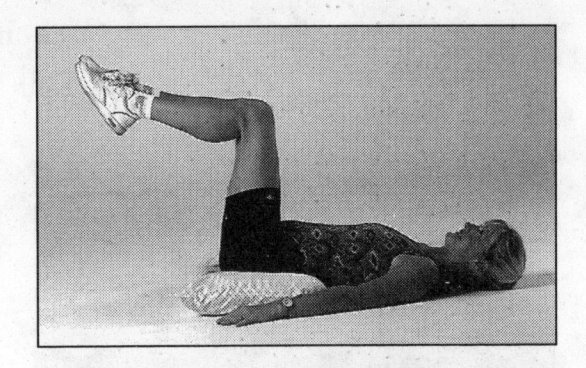

(b) Raise and extend your right leg, toes pointed. Draw your left knee towards your chest, flexing left foot.

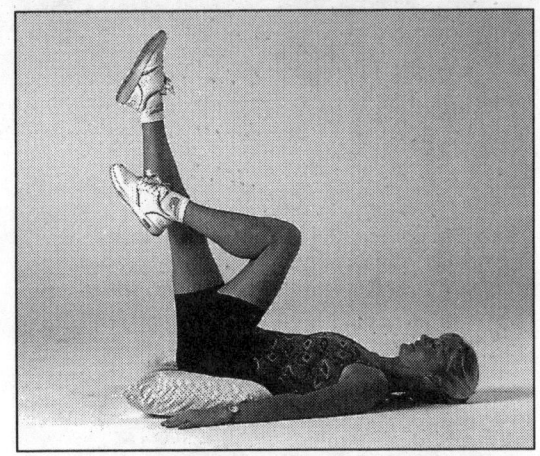

(c) Tuck in your stomach muscles tightly and reverse legs. Draw your right knee towards your chest and flex your right foot, as you extend your left leg. Keep the toes on your left foot pointed as you straighten your left leg. Exhale as you draw knee towards chest, inhale as you reverse legs.

Return to the starting position.

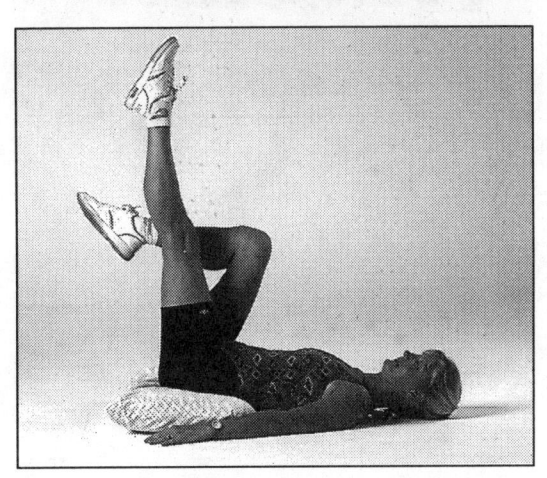

The Double Fat-Burning Exercise Program

Exercise 8: Rope Climbing

Starting position (not shown): lie on floor with knees bent, feet slightly apart, arms at side.

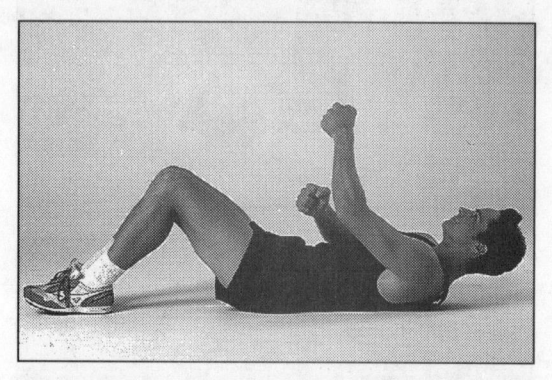

(a) Raise your head and shoulders from floor, pulling yourself up hand over hand with an imaginary rope.

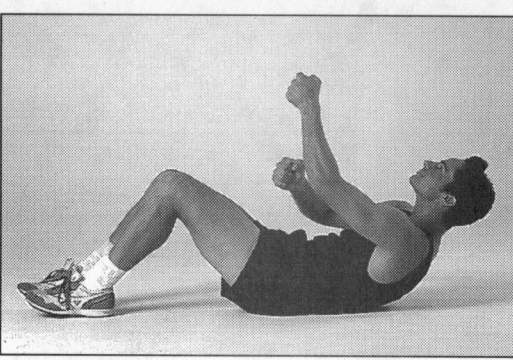

(b) With stomach muscles tucked in tight, continue to lift your upper body off the floor with the rope. Keep your spine curved, not arched.

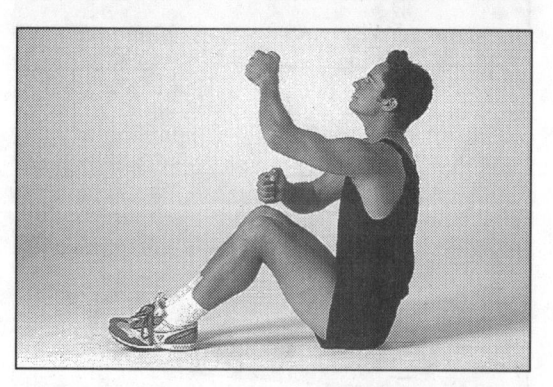

(c) Keep on raising your body, hand over hand, until you are sitting upright.

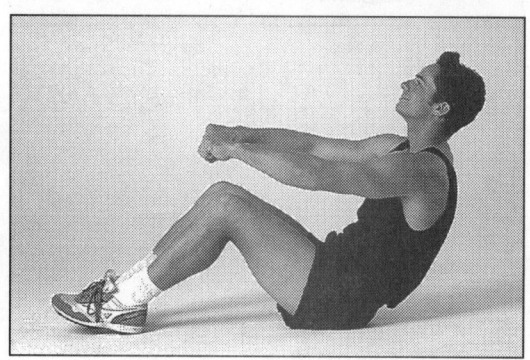

(d) Extend your arms in front at shoulder level, hands balled into fists, and slowly lower your body down to floor. Make sure your stomach muscles are tucked in tight.

Breathe regularly throughout this exercise.

Putting It Together

This book describes the only three effective and safe ways to lose fat. The most effective way is the double fat-burning exercise program, since exercise is the only way to speed up your metabolic rate and thereby burn up more fat. The slowing down of our metabolic rate as we age is the root cause of surplus fat. The exercise program in this book is especially effective because it has a double fat-burning effect. Another marvellous thing about this sort of exercise is that the increase in metabolic rate occurs twenty-four hours a day, even while you are sleeping.

The extra bonus from this exercise program is that you will become fit, have more energy and sleep better.

The second effective way to shed fat is to have a nutritious diet. This does not mean dieting. I have already shown that dieting eventually makes you fatter as well as being detrimental to your health. Basically, a nutritious diet means replacing some of your high fat, high sugar foods (processed food, fast food, junk food), with high complex carbohydrate foods (fruits, vegetables, wholegrains). You don't have to be extreme and give up all your favourite foods. Just reduce the baddies and increase the goodies: your health will certainly improve as well.

How this works is very simple. First, since complex carbohydrates are very nourishing, you will need to eat less of it than low-nourishment foods. Your appetite centre in the brain is satisfied sooner and this results in the cessation of hunger signals. In other words, you are too full to eat junk food. Second, nourishing foods are low in fat and sugar; the two major high kilojoule sources.

The final way to shed fat is to consume most of your kilojoules before 2 p.m. Kilojoules consumed in the first part of the day are burned up more efficiently than those consumed in the latter part. I suggest that for afternoon tea you have a light snack, such as a piece of fruit, and have a light evening meal of protein (fish, meat, eggs, etc.) and vegetables. Stay away from desserts in the evening.

Finally, remember it's taken many years to accumulate the excess fat and your metabolic rate has probably been lowered by previous dieting so it will take a few months to achieve significant fat loss. The change in your lifestyle is worth it—not only will you become slimmer, but you will also feel better, and your health and vitality level will greatly improve.

Recipes to Help You Stay Slim

VEGETABLE RECIPES

Three Rs of cooking vegetables
- Reduce water used (steam the vegetables).
- Reduce length of cooking time.
- Reduce the cut surface area that is exposed to air and water.

How to preserve nutrients in preparation
- Avoid fine shredding, dicing and cutting as much as possible.
- Minimise the number of times mashed or whipped vegetables are served.
- Trim and peel vegetables as little as possible.
- If peeled, avoid excessive peeling to preserve nutrients under the skin.

How to preserve nutrients in cooking
- Avoid stirring air into the vegetables while they are cooking.
- Avoid using soda to brighten vegetables; this destroys B vitamins.
- Serve immediately once cooked.

Vegie Juice
Serves 2

This juice provides a refreshing source of vitamins A and C.

Ingredients
3 ripe tomatoes, chopped
1 cup spinach leaves, chopped
1 clove garlic
1/4 cup of water
black pepper

Method
Blend all ingredients until well combined in a food processor or blender. Season with pepper to taste and serve on ice with a celery swizzle stick.

> *Handy Hint*
> For a spicy flavour, add a few drops of Tabasco sauce.

STEAM COOKING

Steam-baked Vegetables

Place any vegetables of your choice in a baking dish on a rack or on some other means of elevation high enough to keep the vegetables out of water.

Add 1.5 cm hot water in baking dish. Cover and bake at 260°C oven for 20 to 30 minutes.

Cabbage with Caraway Seeds
Serves 4–6

Ingredients
6 cups cabbage, shredded
2 teaspoons margarine (optional)
125 ml (½ cup) skim milk
½ teaspoon caraway seed
½ teaspoon salt

Method
Steam cabbage until just tender (about 4 to 5 minutes). Melt margarine in heated milk. Add cabbage and seasonings and serve.

Carrots with Parsley
Serves 4–6

Ingredients
4 cups carrots, sliced and wedged
½ teaspoon salt
½ cup parsley, minced

Method
Steam carrots 10 to 15 minutes. Mix in salt and parsley and serve.

You may use ¼ cup of dried parsley instead of fresh parsley.

Green Beans with Sesame Seeds
Serves 4

Ingredients
4 cups green beans
2 tablespoons sesame seeds
1/4 cup slivered almonds
1 tablespoon oil
1/2 teaspoon salt
1 teaspoon lemon juice

Method
Steam beans until crispy tender. Lightly brown seeds and almonds in oil. Add salt and lemon juice to sesame seeds and almonds. Mix with green beans.

You do not have to use oil, but make sure you stir frequently if you elect not to.

Minted Peas with Lemon
Serves 4

Ingredients
2 cups peas
1 tablespoon fresh mint, minced (or 2 teaspoons of dry mint)
1 teaspoon lemon peel, grated

Method
Steam peas and mint. Add lemon peel. Toss to coat peas and serve.

Lightly steamed vegetables with a smooth creamy purée make interesting and healthy snacks. Invent your own combinations or try the following.

Steamed Cauliflower with Carrot Purée
Serves 4

Ingredients
4 large cauliflower florets
2 carrots
1 garlic clove
pinch nutmeg
4 tablespoons low-fat milk
2 tablespoons ricotta cheese
freshly ground black pepper

Method
Steam or microwave the cauliflower while you make the purée.

Steam or microwave the carrots until tender. Purée carrots with all remaining ingredients.

Reheat purée gently, if necessary, and pour over cauliflower florets.

Curried Cauliflower
Serves 4–6

Ingredients
1 whole medium cauliflower with leaves removed
1 garlic clove, crushed
2–3 teaspoons curry powder
black pepper

Method
Place whole cauliflower and garlic in a steamer. Steam until tender, about 40 minutes. Serve whole on a platter of cauliflower leaves. Sprinkle with black pepper and rub the top with curry powder. Serve with curries.

Mixed Steamed Vegetables
Serves 4

Ingredients
5 medium carrots, peeled and sliced
2 cups peas
2 leeks cut into thick slices
dash of pepper
chives and poppy seeds

Method
Steam carrots, peas and leeks in a steamer for 20 minutes with lid on. Serve in a small casserole sprinkled with chopped chives, poppy seeds and a dash of black pepper.

STIR-FRIED DISHES

Stir-fried Greens
Serves 2–4

Ingredients
1 tablespoon oil
½ cup onion, thinly sliced*
4 cups greens, washed and drained
½ teaspoon salt

Method
Saute onion in oil until nearly clear and separated into rings. Do not brown.

Pull greens into bite-sized pieces. Do not completely dry them as the moisture aids in the steam-cooking. Add the onions.

Cook for 3 to 5 minutes, stirring constantly.

*You may substitute 1–2 cloves of garlic, minced.

Some Tips for Stir-frying Greens
- Do not heat oil to the smoking stage.
- Cut out the mid-rib and slice it diagonally for greens that have a thick mid-rib such as silverbeet.
- A minimum amount of oil is used in stir-frying so the results should not be greasy.
- Stir-fry vegetables just before the rest of the meal is ready to serve.
- Greens are improved by slightly frying either sliced onion or shallots before adding the greens.
- Vegetables such as green beans, celery and asparagus are best cut diagonally.
- Broccoli stems should be peeled and sliced.
- Vary the seasonings and/or flavour by using any of the following: dill, sweet basil leaves, thyme, oregano leaves, tarragon, soy sauce, mushrooms, slivered almonds, cashews, lemon juice, parsley, garlic, garlic salt, or a sprinkle of Torula yeast.
- Stir-fried vegetables should be served tender and crisp, and green vegetables should be a beautiful green.

Chinese Broccoli
Serves 2–4

Ingredients
2 tablespoons oil
2 tablespoons water
1 tablespoon soy sauce
2 cups broccoli, trimmed and sliced
1 cup celery, thinly sliced
½ cup water chestnuts, drained and sliced
1 tablespoon sesame seeds, toasted

Method
Combine first three ingredients in a large frypan. Heat to boiling. Stir in next three ingredients and heat to boiling again. Cover and steam 5 to 10 minutes or until broccoli is crispy tender. Stir in sesame seeds and serve.

Stir-fry Vegetables
Serves 4

Colourful and crunchy, these vegetables can be served with any meat or fish dish.

Ingredients
1 head broccoli
1 medium red capsicum, cut into thin strips
1 cup fresh mushrooms, sliced
1 tablespoon oil
1 tablespoon soy sauce
1 tablespoon fresh ginger, grated
1 teaspoon cornflour
½ cup water

Method

Heat oil in large frypan or wok. Add garlic, ginger, vegetables and soy sauce to pan. Cook over high heat, stirring for 2 to 3 minutes.

Mix cornflour with water and stir into vegetables until sauce thickens. Serve hot.

Microwave

Preheat browning plate on HIGH for 4 minutes. Add oil, soy sauce, ginger and vegetables. Cover and cook on HIGH for 4 minutes, stirring halfway through cooking. Mix cornflour and water and stir into vegetables. Cook on HIGH 1 to 2 minutes until sauce thickens.

> *Handy Hint*
> For a quick and easy meal, add any leftover meat or seafood pieces to the vegetables during the last 3 to 5 minutes of cooking.

Curried Vegetable and Rice Medley

Serves 4

Cook two or three cups of rice in the conventional way for this recipe.

Ingredients

1 small red pepper	1 teaspoon curry powder
2 carrots	1 teaspoon dried cumin
250 g broccoli	2 tablespoons fruit chutney
2 teaspoons oil	125 g small mushrooms, sliced
1 onion, chopped	1/2 cup water
1 garlic clove, crushed	2 cups cooked rice

Microwave

Cut pepper and carrots into strips, cut broccoli into florets. Combine oil and onion in large shallow dish, cook on HIGH 2 minutes, add garlic, curry powder and cumin, cook on HIGH 1 minute, stir in chutney. Stir in pepper, carrot, mushrooms, broccoli and water, cover, cook on HIGH 5 minutes, or until vegetables are tender. Stir in rice, cook on HIGH 2 minutes or until heated through.

FAMILY MEALS

Stuffed Baked Eggplant
Serves 4

Eggplant (or aubergine) is a meaty vegetable often served in Italian households. Serve this dish as a change from meat.

Ingredients
4 medium eggplants
1 tablespooon olive oil
2 large ripe tomatoes, finely chopped
2 garlic cloves, crushed
4 tablespoons finely chopped parsley

3 cups fresh breadcrumbs
50 g grated parmesan cheese
2 tablespoons finely chopped onion
black pepper to taste

Method
Preheat oven to 200°C. Slice the eggplant in half lengthwise. Scoop out as much of the flesh as you can with a knife—be careful not to pierce the skin. Chop the flesh into cubes and fry in the olive oil until soft. Cool and mix with all other ingredients. Fill eggplant half with mixture and bake for about 40 minutes.

Microwave
Prepare eggplant halves as above. Microwave, covered on HIGH for 20 to 30 minutes or until tender.

Crunchy Vegetable Bake
Serves 4

Choose your favourite vegetable combination for this delicious family meal.

Ingredients
6 cups mixed vegetables, steamed and chopped (choose from carrots, potatoes, pumpkin, onions, leeks, cauliflower, broccoli, turnips, zucchini, celery, cabbage, corn, beans)

1 tablespoon soy sauce
1/2 cup nuts, ground
1/4 cup sesame seeds
2 tablespoons sunflower seeds
1 cup fresh breadcrumbs
2 tablespoons tahini (sesame seed paste)

Method
Preheat oven to 180°C. Combine the vegetables and soy sauce. Pile mixture into a casserole dish. In a bowl, combine remaining ingredients and mix well. Spread topping over vegetables and bake in a moderate oven for 10 to 15 minutes.

Broccoli and Mushroom Pie

Serves 4

Simple but very tasty. Substitute your favourite vegetables. Can be served with extra vegetables or salad for a simple family meal.

Ingredients

500 g potatoes, cooked and mashed
3 cups broccoli florets
3 cups mushrooms, finely sliced
1 small onion, finely chopped
4 tablespoons light cream cheese
parmesan cheese

Method

Steam or microwave the broccoli and mushrooms until just tender. While they are still hot, stir in onion, cream cheese and pepper to taste. Place in shallow ovenproof dish or four individual dishes. Cover with mashed potato, smooth with a fork. Sprinkle with parmesan cheese. Place under hot grill until golden brown.

Serve hot.

Pumpkin Bake

Serves 4

Healthy and wholesome, this would be perfect with a roast dinner.

Ingredients

500 g pumpkin, peeled and sliced very thinly
$1/2$ onion, finely chopped
2 teaspoons cornflour
1 cup low-fat milk
1 tablespoon parmesan cheese

Method

Stir cornflour into milk. Add onion and bring to the boil. Stir until sauce is thickened.

Toss sauce with pumpkin and place in shallow baking dish. Sprinkle with parmesan cheese and bake in moderate oven for 35 to 40 minutes, or until pumpkin is tender.

Microwave

Place layers of pumpkin in a microwave-safe casserole dish, with 1 tablespoon of water. Cover and cook on HIGH for 6 minutes. Mix cornflour, milk and onion and toss with pumpkin. Cover and cook on HIGH for 1 to 2 minutes until sauce begins to thicken. Sprinkle with parmesan cheese and cook uncovered on HIGH for a further 1 to 2 minutes.

Cabbage Rolls
Serves 6

Ingredients
12 large cabbage leaves

Filling
1 medium onion, diced
1/2 teaspoon ginger, finely chopped
2 tablespoons water
600 g lean minced beef or veal
1/2 teaspoon cumin
1 teaspoon coriander
1 carrot, grated
1/2 zucchini
2 cups cooked brown rice

Easy Tomato Sauce
6 large, ripe tomatoes, roughly chopped
1/2 cup white wine or water
1/2 onion, chopped
3 tablespoons tomato paste
1 garlic clove, crushed
2 tablespoons fresh parsley

Place all ingredients in a small saucepan and cook on medium heat for about 15 minutes (or microwave in covered dish on HIGH for 5 minutes).

Method
Steam cabbage leaves until tender. Drain and cool.

In a saucepan, combine onion, ginger and water. Cover and cook until onion softens. Add meat and spices and cook until meat is done. Stir in carrot, zucchini and rice and mix well.

Divide mixture among the 12 cabbage leaves and carefully roll up, securing each end. Place side by side in an ovenproof dish, pour Easy Tomato Sauce and bake at 200°C for 15 to 20 minutes, or until all ingredients are heated through. Serve hot with steamed carrots and potatoes.

Microwave
Cook cabbage leaves six at a time on a large glass platter. Microwave 6 minutes on HIGH or until cabbage leaves are tender and can be folded over. Repeat with remaining six cabbage leaves.

Place onion, ginger and water in a small casserole. Cover. Microwave 5 minutes on HIGH. Stir. Add meat and break up. Microwave 10 minutes on HIGH. Break up meat halfway through cooking. Add all other ingredients and mix well. Divide evenly among the 12 cabbage leaves. Carefully roll up, being sure to secure each end. Place six cabbage rolls in a baking dish (approx. 20 cm × 30 cm). Repeat with remaining six cabbage rolls.

Divide sauce evenly and pour over top of cabbage rolls. Cover baking dish with plastic wrap. Microwave on HIGH for 10 to 12 minutes or until cabbage rolls are heated through.

Handy Hints
This recipe also serves 12 as a light entrée. Also, to remove cabbage leaves easily, let cold water run underneath each leaf until the weight of the water makes them fall away easily.

Vegetarian Stuffed Cabbage Leaves

Ingredients
8 large cabbage leaves
1/2 cup onion, chopped
1 cup celery, chopped
1/2 cup sweet corn kernels or fresh corn
3 mushrooms, chopped
1 cup wholemeal breadcrumbs
1/2 teaspoon thyme

Method
Wash cabbage leaves and cook for 5 minutes in water until tender. Retain water. Sauté mushrooms and onion for 2 minutes. Add the other ingredients and mix well. Place a spoonful of the mixture on each leaf and roll up to make little parcels. Cook in the cabbage water for 20 minutes.

Chinese Vegetables in Satay Sauce
Serves 4

Ingredients
30 g Chinese dried mushrooms
1 tablespoon oil
1 teaspoon grated fresh ginger
200 g snow peas, topped and tailed
1 red pepper, chopped
425 g can baby corn cuts, drained
1 1/2 tablespoons cornflour
1 cup chicken stock
2 teaspoons satay sauce
2 cups (125 g) bean sprouts
2 green shallots, chopped

Microwave
Place mushrooms in small bowl, cover with hot water, cook on HIGH 5 minutes or until mushrooms are soft. Stand 5 minutes, drain, discard stalks, chop caps roughly.

Combine oil, ginger, snow peas and pepper in deep dish, cook on HIGH 4 minutes or until vegetables begin to soften. Add mushrooms, corn, blended cornflour and stock and satay sauce to vegetables. Cook on HIGH 3 minutes or until mixture boils and thickens, stirring occasionally. Stir in bean sprouts and shallots, heat on HIGH 1 minute.

Instant Vegetarian Pizza
Serves 2–3

Ingredients
2 rounds Lebanese flat bread
2 tablespoons tomato paste
3 medium tomatoes, peeled, sliced
1 large new potato, grated
1 onion, chopped
1 red pepper, chopped
125 g small mushrooms
10 stuffed olives, sliced
250 g mozzarella cheese, grated
2 tablespoons grated parmesan cheese

Microwave
Spread bread with tomato paste, top with tomato, then potato. Sprinkle with onion, pepper, mushrooms and olives. Sprinkle with combined

cheeses, cook one at a time on HIGH 8 minutes or until potato is tender and cheese melted.

Leek and Vegetable Casserole
Serves 4

Ingredients
6 large leeks, washed and sliced into 2.5 cm cubes, leaving about 2.5 cm of the green part
2 large potatoes, peeled and thinly sliced
2 medium carrots, chopped
1 1/2 cups stock of choice
1/2 cabbage, shredded
black pepper

Method
Layer leeks, potatoes, carrots and cabbage in a casserole dish. Repeat this sequence, end with cabbage. Pour stock over vegetable layers, sprinkle with black pepper. Bake in a moderate oven about 30 minutes or until cooked. Serve with steamed corn kernels cut into 5 cm chunks, stuffed tomatoes and side salad.

Baked Eggplant with Cottage Cheese Sauce
Serves 3–4

Ingredients
2 large eggplants
1 large onion, chopped
3 tomatoes, chopped
1 teaspoon basil
1 tablespoon parsley, chopped
1 teaspoon black pepper
1 teaspoon soy sauce, low salt
3/4 cup non-fat cottage cheese
2–3 tablespoons milk
2 tablespoons dry wholemeal breadcrumbs

Methods
Wash eggplants, don't peel. Cut into 1 cm slices. Brown in a non-stick frypan. Set aside slices. In the same pan, sauté onion, tomatoes, basil, parsley, black pepper and soy sauce in a little water for 10 minutes.

Blend cottage cheese and milk together. Divide eggplant slices into three portions. Place one portion in a casserole, top with half tomato mixture and spread half cheese sauce on top of tomato. Place on more eggplant slices, then remaining tomato mixture and cheese sauce. Finish with a layer of eggplant. Top with breadcrumbs. Bake 175°C for about 20 minutes.

Ratatouille
Serves 4

Ingredients
1 eggplant, chopped
2 green peppers, chopped
2 garlic cloves, crushed
1/2 teaspoon oregano
2 zucchini, sliced
12 button onions, peeled
12 cherry tomatoes

Method
Combine ingredients, add a little water, cook over low heat to prevent sticking, about 30 minutes.

Vegetable Paella
Serves 4

Ingredients
1 1/4 cups brown rice
2 cups chicken stock
2 large onions, sliced
3 large carrots, diced
3 zucchini, sliced thick
2 garlic cloves
3 tomatoes
1 red pepper
1 green pepper
1 tablespoon tomato paste
1/2 teaspoon turmeric
pepper
250 g broccoli

Method
Parboil rice in stock for 15 minutes, set aside. Add sliced onions, diced carrots, thickly sliced zucchini and crushed garlic to a non-stick frypan and cook about 10 minutes in 3 tablespoons water over medium heat. Add seeded and sliced peppers, tomato paste, turmeric and chopped tomatoes (peeled), cook for further 2 minutes. Add rice with stock and pepper (if desired) and stir until well combined with the rest. Simmer gently for further 15 minutes.

Separately boil florets of broccoli for 3 minutes, drain and add to the rest. Arrange paella on serving plate and garnish with lemon wedges.

Rice and Lentil Casserole
Serves 4

Ingredients
1 cup lentils
2 cups water
1 chopped onion
1/8 teaspoon chilli powder
1 cup rice
1 cup chopped tomatoes
1 garlic clove, crushed
cayenne pepper

Method
In a saucepan bring lentils and rice to boil. Reduce heat and simmer 1 to 1 1/2 hours. Add tomatoes, onion, garlic, chilli powder and cayenne. Place in

a baking dish. Bake covered for 20 minutes. Sprinkle sapsago cheese on top and bake uncovered 10 minutes.

Spanish Rice
Serves 4

Ingredients
2 cups cooked brown rice
2 cups chopped fresh tomatoes
2 onions, chopped
¼ cup chopped celery
1 garlic clove, crushed
2 teaspoons soy sauce, low salt
½ teaspoon chilli powder
⅛ teaspoon ground cumin
1 green pepper, sliced

Method
Simmer the tomatoes, onions, celery, garlic, soy sauce, chilli powder and cumin 10 to 15 minutes, until tender. Add the green pepper and cook 2 to 3 minutes. Stir in the rice, heat and serve.

Samosas (Hot Vegetable Curry Pastries)
Makes approximately 36 triangles

Ingredients
1 small onion, finely chopped
3 florets cauliflower, chopped
1 tablespoon butter
2 small potatoes, cooked and cut into small cubes
½ cup frozen peas
2 teaspoons garam masala or curry powder
1 tablespoon chopped fresh parsley
1 teaspoon fresh mint
1 tablespoon lemon juice
1 pack (25 cm) frozen spring-roll wrappers, thawed

Method
Lightly fry the onion and cauliflower in the butter until coloured. Add the potatoes and peas and gently fry for 2 minutes, stir in remaining ingredients (except spring-roll wrappers). Mix well, simmer for 1 to 2 minutes, spoon onto a plate, chill and set aside until required.

Separate the spring-roll wrappers and cut into strips 4.5 cm wide.

To fill pastries—place 1 to 2 teaspoons of the filling onto one end of the pastry strip, fold over keeping a triangular shape and seal the edges; continue folding pastry over so that filling is wrapped in a triangular parcel. Brush with cold water and ensure edges are well sealed.

Wipe out wok or deep fry pan with absorbent kitchen paper, add enough cooking oil to fill the wok one-third full. Heat until hot (220°C; this is when a 2 cm cube of bread will turn crisply brown in just 30 seconds).

Deep-fry the pastries, six at a time, until golden brown. Lift out carefully with a draining spoon and rest for 1 to 2 minutes on absorbent kitchen paper before serving.

SOUPS

Pumpkin and Parsnip Soup
Serves 8

A tasty soup special enough to serve at a dinner party.

Ingredients
800 g pumpkin, peeled and chopped
2 large parsnips, peeled and chopped
4 cups chicken stock (see below) or water and stock cubes
½ teaspoon freshly grated nutmeg
6 tablespoons coconut milk, available canned in supermarkets

Method
Place pumpkin, parsnips and chicken stock or water and stock cubes in large saucepan and bring to the boil. Cover and cook until tender. Purée in processor or blender until smooth. Reheat, add nutmeg and coconut milk. Serve hot. Add more water for a thinner soup.

Microwave
Place the pumpkin and parsnips in a 3–4 litre casserole dish with one cup of stock. Cover and cook on HIGH for 10 minutes or until tender. Continue as above.

Spring Vegetable Soup
Serves 4

This is a clear soup scattered with finely chopped vegetables. A good chicken stock is required.

Ingredients

Chicken stock

2 kg chicken bones
2 onions
2 carrots
1 stick celery
1 tablespoon peppercorns
8 litres water

Method
Place all ingredients in a large saucepan, bring to the boil and simmer uncovered for 2 to 3 hours. Skim often. Strain and refrigerate overnight. Remove all traces of fat. Proceed with soup recipe.

Ingredients
2 carrots, peeled and sliced into thin sticks
1 stick celery, sliced into thin sticks
10 runner beans, topped, tailed and sliced into thin strips
100 g mushrooms, finely sliced
1 punnet cherry tomatoes
2 tablespoons fresh parsley, finely chopped

Method
Place carrots, celery, beans and mushrooms into boiling stock, cook 5 minutes. Add cherry tomatoes and parsley. Cook a further 1 minute and serve hot.

> **Handy Hint**
> Chop the carrots, celery and beans to the same size. For a more substantial soup, add shredded chicken or a few prawns and some finely sliced snow peas and spring onion.

Hearty Vegetable Soup
Serves 6

Ingredients
6 cups vegetable stock
2 onions, chopped
2 garlic cloves, crushed
4 celery stalks, chopped
3 carrots, diced
½ turnip, chopped
1 parsnip, chopped

2 potatoes, chopped
1 sweet potato, chopped
½ cup green peas
½ cup fresh corn kernels
2 tablespoons tomato paste (unsalted)
1 teaspoon soy sauce, low salt

Method
Add all ingredients except peas and corn to stock. Simmer 20 minutes, add peas and corn and simmer further 10 minutes. Garnish with chopped parsley and alfalfa sprouts.

To make a stew, use less water and thicken with wholemeal flour.

Lentil Vegetable Soup
Serves 8–10

Ingredients
8 cups water
2 cups dry lentils, washed
½ cup onion, chopped
½ cup celery, diced
½ cup carrots, diced

½ cup potatoes, diced
½ cup spinach, shredded
1 garlic clove, minced
½ teaspoon oregano

Method
Combine all ingredients in a large saucepan and simmer 30 to 45 minutes or until cooked.

Microwave
Place lentils, vegetables and seasoning in a 3–4 litre casserole dish with 2 cups of water. Cover and microwave on MEDIUM-HIGH for 15 minutes. Add the remaining stock and heat through.

Red Lentil Soup
Serves 4

Ingredients

2½ cups red lentils
2½ cups chicken stock
1 onion, chopped
2 garlic cloves, crushed
2 tomatoes, skinned
1 bay leaf
½ teaspoon oregano
1 teaspoon cider vinegar or lemon juice

Method

Soak lentils in water overnight. Rinse, cover with chicken stock, add onion, garlic, tomatoes, bay leaf and oregano. Bring to boil, cover and simmer for 35 minutes. Add vinegar. Garnish with parsley and twisted lemon.

Cauliflower Soup
Serves 4

Ingredients

2 cups chicken stock
½ cauliflower, chopped into pieces
2 garlic cloves, peeled
¼–½ cup sour cream
1 cup skim milk
1 teaspoon non-fat dry milk blended with skim milk
sapsago cheese, parsley and paprika

Method

Place cauliflower, stock and garlic in a saucepan. Cook for 30 minutes until tender. Put mixture into a blender, add skim milk to required thickness. Add sour cream and heat. Garnish with cheese, parsley and paprika.

Tomato Soup
Serves 4

Ingredients

6 ripe juicy tomatoes, peeled and chopped or salt-free canned tomatoes
2 cups vegetable or chicken stock
2 tablespoons tomato paste
1 small carrot, chopped
1 stalk celery, chopped
1 small onion, chopped
2 garlic cloves, chopped
1 tablespoon cornflour blended with water
black pepper
1 bay leaf
1 clove
½ teaspoon oregano

Method

Sauté carrot, celery, onion and garlic in a little of the stock. Add remaining stock, tomatoes, pepper and herbs. Blend in tomato paste and cornflour. Cook slowly for 30 minutes. Cool. Take out clove and bay leaf, put soup through a sieve or electric blender. Serve with chopped parsley and croutons and add a dash of sour cream or lemon juice.

Add ½ cup cooked brown rice to make a thicker soup or you can make cream of tomato soup by adding 1 cup of stock and 1 cup of milk.

SALAD RECIPES

To get the best from your salad simply:
- Choose contrasting texture, colour, form and flavour in selecting ingredients.
- Use chilled plates or bowls in serving to keep ingredients cool and crisp.
- Select various salad greens and combine several in the same salad.
- Be generous when slicing or chunking salad ingredients.
- Break or tear greens by hand into bite-size pieces rather than cutting them with a knife.
- A salad fork and spoon work the best in tossing a salad.
- Toss using a rolling motion—do not stir.

Select the correct dressing
- Tangy oil-herb dressings go nicely with greens or they can be used for marinating vegetables.
- Salad dressing is a natural for potato salad or moulded salads.
- For a zippy dressing that adds flavour to fruit salads and substitutes for sour cream, mix yoghurt or buttermilk with lemon juice and a small pinch of salt.
- Use a minimum of dressing; besides adding kilojoules, too much dressing makes a limp, dripping salad.
- For some salads, all you need do is add a little seasoned salt and/or lemon juice.
- For salads containing greens, add the dressing at the last moment.

To garnish a salad attractively:
- Any colour contrast with a complementary flavour adds spark to a salad, but remember not to overdo it.
- Try a sliver of olive, a sprig of watercress or mint, fresh strawberries, a wedge of apple or tomato, a slice of beetroot, a carrot curl, parsley, paprika or what about onion rings, celery fans, or avocado slices.

Tomato and Cucumber Salad
Serves 4

Ingredients
2 cups tomato, sliced
2 cups cucumber, sliced
1½ cups onion rings
¼ cup lemon juice

Method
Combine all ingredients and chill for at least 15 to 20 minutes.

Tossed Salad with Avocado
Serves 6

Ingredients
3 cups lettuce pieces, torn
3 cups spinach pieces, torn
1 medium cucumber, sliced
1½ cups tomato pieces
3 spring onions, chopped
1 medium avocado, sliced
½ cup radish, sliced
½ cup pitted black olives, sliced
seasoned salt to taste
lemon juice to taste

Method
Combine all ingredients and toss just before serving!

Avocado Green Salad
Serves 2

Ingredients
2 lettuce leaves
1 large avocado, sliced
½ cup bean sprouts
2 tablespoons lemon-garlic dressing (below)

Method
Place avocado on lettuce leaves. Sprinkle sprouts on top. Cover with lemon-garlic dressing.

Lemon-Garlic Dressing
Makes ½ cup

Ingredients
¼ cup lemon juice
¼ cup sesame oil
¼ cup sesame seeds, toasted
1 garlic clove, crushed

Method
Blend lemon juice and oil and add sesame seeds and garlic. Store this dressing in the refrigerator.

Rice Salad
Serves 4

Ingredients
2 cups brown rice, cooked
½ cup peas, cooked
2 tablespoons sunflower seed kernels
½ cup corn niblets
¼ cup red capsicum, minced
1 tablespoon chives, chopped
¼ cup smoke-flavoured textured vegetable protein (optional)

Method
Rehydrate the textured vegetable protein (TVP) in 60 ml (¼ cup) hot water. Combine all ingredients. Serve.

Speedy Bean Salad
Serves 4

Ingredients
1 cup four-bean mix, drained
1 cup cut baby corn, drained
¾ cup bean sprouts
2 tablespoons lemon-garlic dressing (see page 148)

Method
Combine the beans, corn and sprouts then mix in dressing. Chill and serve.

Coleslaw
Serves 6

Ingredients
1 cup four-bean mix, drained
4 cups cabbage, shredded
½ cup capsicum, chopped finely
¼ cup chives, chopped
⅓ cup lemon-garlic dressing (see page 148)

Method
Combine all ingredients. Add lemon-garlic dressing and toss. Chill and serve.

You may add or substitute with one cup of baby corn, one cup of shredded spinach, one cup pineapple pieces, one cup of sliced zucchini, one cup of chopped nuts or one cup of grated carrot.

Oriental Salad
Serves 4

Ingredients
1 cup cauliflower, broken into tiny florets
2 cups cabbage, shredded
1 cup bean shoots
½ green capsicum, finely sliced
½ red capsicum, finely sliced
½ carrot, finely sliced
2 tablespoons sesame seeds
1 cup shredded lettuce
1 quantity low-fat Oriental Dressing (see recipe)

Method
Toss all ingredients along with Oriental dressing.

Handy Hint
Turn into a main meal by adding two cups shredded cooked chicken or beef.

Low-Fat Oriental Salad Dressing

Ingredients
2 tablespoons soy sauce, low salt
1 garlic clove, crushed
1 teaspoon sesame oil
1 teaspoon honey

Method
Combine all ingredients and mix thoroughly.

Grilled Eggplant and Tomato Salad
Serves 4

Add some mozzarella, feta or low-fat cheese to this dish and you have a delicious entrée or light meal.

Ingredients
1 medium eggplant
2 large firm but ripe tomatoes
1 tablespoon olive oil
fresh parsley or basil leaves for garnish

Method
Slice the eggplant into eight thin round slices. Brush both sides of eggplant with olive oil and grill under hot grill until cooked and browned on each side. Turn once. Slice tomatoes and arrange with eggplant on serving dish. Garnish with parsley or basil.

Curried Egg Salad
Serves 6–8

Ingredients
8 eggs
2 sticks celery
4 shallots
3 tablespoons chopped parsley
6 thin slices square white bread
60 g butter
3 tablespoons grated parmesan cheese
lettuce leaves

Method
Put eggs into saucepan of cold water. Cover and bring to boil then reduce heat and simmer for 8 to 10 minutes. Drain off hot water and cover with cold water. Shell eggs when cold. Mix thinly sliced celery, chopped shallots and parsley in a bowl. Remove crusts from bread and cut each slice into three rounds using 4 cm cutter. Place rounds on an oven tray; brush each side with melted butter; sprinkle over parmesan cheese. Bake in moderate oven 10 minutes or until golden brown; cool.

Line serving plate with lettuce leaves. Arrange halved eggs on one side of plate, spoon celery mixture beside eggs, then place bread rounds next to celery mixture. Refrigerate until ready to serve. Serve curry mayonnaise separately.

Curry Mayonnaise

Ingredients
1 medium onion
60 g butter
1 tablespoon curry powder
½ cup mayonnaise
1 tablespoon lemon juice
½ cup light cream
salt and pepper to taste

Method
Heat butter in pan and add peeled and finely chopped onion. Sauté gently until onion is transparent; add curry powder and cook 1 minute. Set aside this mixture until it is cold then combine it with the mayonnaise, lemon juice, salt and pepper. Beat cream until soft peaks form and fold into mayonnaise mixture.

Italian Mixed Salad
Serves 6

Ingredients
125 g green beans
125 g button mushrooms
12 small onions
1 green pepper
2 carrots
1 small cauliflower
1 small eggplant
2 sticks celery
¼ cup oil

Dressing
½ cup bottled Italian dressing
1 garlic clove
2 teaspoons prepared mustard

Method
Trim and string beans, cut into 5 cm lengths. Trim mushrooms then peel and quarter onions. Remove stalk from pepper and cut into strips. Peel carrots and cut diagonally into 2.5 cm chunks. Divide cauliflower into florets. Cut unpeeled eggplant into 2.5 cm cubes and cut celery diagonally into 2.5 cm slices. Sauté vegetables in hot oil for 5 minutes then transfer into a large salad bowl. Add dressing and toss lightly.

Dressing
Combine all ingredients in screw-top jar, shake well.

Italian Prawn Salad
Serves 4 as an entrée or luncheon dish

Ingredients
500 g cooked prawns
2 tomatoes
470 g can artichoke hearts
60 g sliced salami
60 g black olives
lettuce leaves

Dressing
1/3 cup lemon juice
1 teaspoon prepared mustard
1 tablespoon chopped parsley

Method
Shell prawns, remove black vein and cut the prawns in half if large. Remove stems from tomatoes, cut into quarters. Drain artichoke hearts, cut in half. Combine prawns, tomato quarters, artichoke pieces, salami and black olives in bowl, toss to combine. Spoon mixture onto lettuce leaves. Before serving, spoon dressing over.

Dressing
Combine all ingredients in screw-top jar. Shake well.

Greek Salad
Serves 6–8

Ingredients
1 small red pepper
1 small green pepper
1 large onion
125 g black olives
2 ripe tomatoes
2 sticks celery
1 cucumber
1 small lettuce
125 g feta cheese
1/4 cup French dressing

Method
Cut red and green peppers into rings, remove any seeds. Peel onion, cut into wedges, separate into pieces. Cut tomatoes into wedges, slice the celery and cut the cucumber into cubes. Wash and dry lettuce, tear into pieces. Put all the prepared vegetables into a salad bowl and add olives. Cover and refrigerate until ready to serve. Add salad dressing, toss well, top salad with sliced feta cheese.

Hot Potato Salad
Serves 6

Ingredients
1 kg potatoes
2 sticks celery
1 onion
1/2 red pepper
2 tablespoons chopped parsley
1/4 cup sour cream
1/3 cup French dressing
salt and pepper
2 rashers bacon
2 hard-boiled eggs
90 g cheese

Method

Peel and dice potatoes, cook in boiling salted water until tender, drain well. Slice celery diagonally, peel and finely chop onion, slice red pepper. Combine hot potatoes, celery, onion, pepper and parsley in a bowl. Mix sour cream and dressing until smooth and season with salt and pepper. Pour the dressing over the potato mixture, mix lightly, spoon into shallow ovenproof dish. Dice bacon and sauté in a pan until crisp. Drain, sprinkle over top of potatoes with chopped eggs. Grate cheese, sprinkle over top of bacon and eggs, then heat the dish under a hot griller until cheese has melted and is golden brown.

Curried Seafood Salad
Serves 6

Ingredients

1½ cups long-grain rice
500 g cooked prawns
500 g scallops
60 g butter
2 sticks celery
2 tablespoons chopped parsley
3 shallots
1 small red pepper
½ cup French dressing
2 teaspoons curry powder
1 teaspoon turmeric
2 teaspoons lemon juice
salt and pepper

Method

Gradually add rice to a large quantity of boiling salted water and boil uncovered 12 minutes or until rice is tender, drain. Spread rice out on flat tray and leave 2 hours or until rice is dry. Shell prawns, remove black vein. Heat butter in a pan, add scallops, cook gently, stirring 3 to 5 minutes or until scallops are tender; drain. Place rice in large bowl, add prawns, scallops, finely chopped celery, parsley, chopped shallots, seeded and finely chopped pepper; toss lightly.

Combine French dressing, curry powder, turmeric, lemon juice and sugar in a bowl, season with salt and pepper. Add dressing to rice mixture and toss thoroughly. Refrigerate until ready to serve.

SPROUT RECIPES

Sprouts are tiny young shoots that emerge from legumes, seeds or grains on the way to becoming mature plants. Some of the most popular are:
Legumes—soy beans, mung beans, lentils, chick peas (garbanzos) and peas
Seeds—sunflower, alfalfa, radish
Grains—wheat, barley, millet, oats, rice, corn and rye.

All sprouts contain high levels of vitamins in the B complex group and vitamins A, C and E. Sprouts also provide fresh greens for salads all year round and they make an inexpensive taste change for your salads.

You may use sprouts for salads, garnishes, main dishes, soups, breads, sandwiches, sweets, waffles and beverages.

How To Grow Sprouts:

- Select a wide-mouth litre jar.
- Select good quality seeds. Use 1/2 cup of medium-sized seeds (mung beans) or 1 tablespoon of fine seeds (alfalfa).
- Wash the seed and place in the jar. Cover with lukewarm water—2 cups for medium-sized seeds and 1/4 cup for fine seeds. Soak overnight.
- Cover the jar opening with cheesecloth or a clean nylon stocking and secure with a rubber band.
- Drain and rinse twice a day for 2–5 days. Distribute seed over the bottom and sides of the jar by shaking. Lay the jar on its side in a warm, dark place, such as a cupboard.
- Sprouts are ready when the sprout is equal in length to the original seed or: alfalfa—2.5–5 cm long; mung beans—4–7.5 cm long; lentils—2.5 cm long
- To develop the green chlorophyll in sprouts, place on a sunlit windowsill for 3–12 hours.
- Cover the jar with a lid and then put it in the refrigerator. The sprouts will keep for several days, like other fresh vegetables.

Beansprout Salad
Serves 6

Ingredients
4 cups bean sprouts, crisped
4 cups spinach, torn and crisped
2 cups tomato pieces
1/4 cup sesame dressing (below)

Method
Combine the first three ingredients. Add dressing. Toss gently and serve.

Sesame Dressing
Makes ½ cup

Ingredients
¼ cup lemon juice
¼ cup sesame oil
¼ cup sesame seeds, toasted

Method
Blend lemon juice and oil. Add sesame seeds. Store in refrigerator.

Alfalfa Garden Salad
Serves 4–6

Ingredients
1 cup alfalfa sprouts, loosely packed
½ cup sunflower seed kernels, toasted
2 cups salad greens, torn and crisped
6 radishes, sliced
½ medium cucumber, sliced
1 tablespoon sesame oil
1 tablespoon lemon juice
⅛ teaspoon salt

Method
Combine the first three ingredients. Blend the last three ingredients and then add to salad. Toss gently and serve.

POTATO RECIPES

Chippies
Serves 4

Everyone loves potato chips. Try them baked in the oven for a low-fat version of this popular snack.

Ingredients
4 medium potatoes, washed with a soft brush to remove any surface dirt

Method
Peel and chop potatoes into chunks, place in very hot oven until golden brown and cooked through, approximately 40 minutes.

Sweet Potato and Leek Pie
Serves 4–6

This unusual rectangular pie is made by alternating layers of filo with the delicious filling.

Ingredients
200 g filo pastry sheets
800 g sweet potato, cooked and chopped into cubes
1 leek, sliced
2 cups low-fat milk
2 tablespoons flour
1 tablespoon mustard powder
1 teaspoon ground cinnamon
2 egg whites, lightly beaten

Method

Mix flour and a little milk to make a smooth paste. Place leek and remaining milk in a small saucepan. Bring to the boil. Remove from heat. Add blended flour. Stir well. Return to the boil stirring constantly.

Add mustard and cinnamon, stir into sweet potato. Allow to cool then mash roughly.

Cut the pastry sheets with scissors to fit a medium size baking dish or tray. Brush oil onto the bottom sides of the dish. Brush alternate layers of filo with egg white until a third of the pastry is used. Spread half the sweet potato mixture on this and continue layers until pastry and filling are used.

Finish by brushing top with egg white. Bake for 35 to 40 minutes, until top is golden brown.

Handy Hints
Can be served with tomato sauce. (See Easy Tomato Sauce recipe, page 139.) Sprinkle top with sesame seeds or parmesan cheese before baking.

Curried Potatoes
Serves 4

This tasty side dish will add zing to a simple grilled fish or meat main course.

Ingredients
1 teaspoon Madras curry powder (or to taste)
4 tablespoons coconut milk (canned)
4 medium potatoes, cut into quarters
1 cup cauliflower florets
1 cup cabbage, chopped
½ onion, chopped
1 cup shelled peas
1 cup water

Method
Place potato, water, curry powder and coconut milk in medium saucepan. Cover, bring to the boil and simmer until potatoes are nearly cooked.

Add cauliflower, cover and cook for a further 5 minutes. Add cabbage, onion and peas and cook 2 to 3 minutes. Add more water if necessary. Potatoes will become a little mushy when ready to serve. Serve hot.

Hot Potato Bean Salad
Serves 4–6

Ingredients
500 g potatoes, thinly sliced
1 large apple, sliced
250 mL carton apple juice
440 g can red kidney beans, drained
3 green shallots, chopped

Microwave
Place potato and apple slices into shallow dish, pour over apple juice, cover, cook on HIGH 5 minutes or until potatoes are tender. Stir in beans, heat on HIGH 3 minutes, sprinkle with shallots.

Italian Potatoes
Serves 6

Ingredients
6 potatoes, peeled and chopped
1 garlic clove, crushed
freshly ground black pepper
2 tomatoes, peeled and chopped
1 teaspoon oregano

Method
Boil potatoes for 30 minutes or until tender. Mash. Beat in remaining ingredients. Serve hot or cold.

Parsley New Potatoes
Serves 3–4

Ingredients
12 small new potatoes
2 tablespoons chopped parsley
1 egg white, beaten

Method
Boil potatoes for 20 minutes or until cooked. Lightly brush with egg white and roll in finely chopped parsley. Place in casserole and heat in oven for 10 minutes.

Spiced Sweet Potato
Serves 4

Ingredients
4 sweet potatoes, approximately 1 kg
1 teaspoon cinnamon
$1/2$ teaspoon ginger
$1/2$ teaspoon nutmeg
1 cup skim milk

Method
Boil the potatoes until they are soft, peel and mash. Stir in spices and add about 1 cup milk. Turn the mixture into a casserole and bake in oven 200°C for 15 minutes. The potatoes may be further flavoured with grated orange peel, or chopped parsley sprinkled over top.

Potato Cakes
Serves 2

Ingredients
2 large potatoes, peeled
1 tablespoon flour
2 egg whites
1 tablespoon milk

Method
Grate potatoes, add egg whites, flour and a little milk. Place spoonful of mixture into frypan. Cook about 7 minutes on each side. Serve with lemon and garlic dressing or cider vinegar.

Sweet Potato Soufflé
Serves 5

Ingredients
3 cups mashed sweet potato
1 cup mashed squash
1 cup skim milk
1 teaspoon powdered skim milk
1 tablespoon lemon juice
$1/2$ teaspoon nutmeg
$1/3$ teaspoon cinnamon
$1/2$ teaspoon ground ginger
1 teaspoon grated lemon or orange rind
3 egg whites, stiffly beaten until peaks form
$2/3$ cup rolled oats

Method
Blend powdered and skim milk. Combine sweet potato, squash and skim milk, add spices, lemon juice and rind. Blend egg whites into potato mixture. Soak oatmeal quickly in cold water to soften, then lay in the bottom of a non-stick baking pan or foil-lined pan. Bake in oven 175°C for 15 minutes or until the oatmeal layer is browned and dry. Fill the pan with sweet potato mixture. Bake for 30 minutes.

Further Reading

Barnard, A., *A Physician's Slimming Guide for Permanent Weight Control,* The Book Publishing Company, New York, 1992.

Cooper, K., *The Aerobics Program for Total Wellbeing,* Bantam Books, New York, 1982.

David, M., *Nourishing Wisdom,* Bell Tower Books, New York, 1991.

Forcyt, J. *Living Without Dieting,* Harrison Publishing, New York, 1992.

Galbraith, P., *Reversing Ageing,* Lothian Books, Melbourne, 1993.

Gittleman, A., *Beyond Pritikin,* Bantam Books, New York, 1989.

Moteljan, G. *Cooking Without Fat,* Health Valley Foods, New York, 1992.

The Weekend Australian Review, 'Exercise Your Right to Never Say Diet', March 21-22, Sydney, 1992.

Time Life Books, *The Fat Body,* Amsterdam, 1987.

Index

aerobic exercise 40
   benefits 44–7
aerobics 55
ageing 47
alcohol 27, 103
appetite-control 38, 99
aspartame 104
attitude, positive 25, 29

bathroom scales 16
brain function 77
bread 96, 100
breakfast 87, 91
butter 84, 101
buttocks 37, 118–119

carbohydrates, complex 74–5
cereals 96
chair-stepping 58
cheese 84
chilli 97
cooling down 53
cycling 55

diet books 22
dieting 86
   positive attitude 25
   rebound 21
   yo-yo 21
diets 7
   failure of 18–19
   health problems 23–4
double fat-burning exercises 41, 43, 48, 55–61

enzymes 44
evening meal 91, 103
exercise
   best time 50, 56
   buttocks 118–119
   causes fat loss 42
   correct 40
   double fat-burning 55–61
   duration 49, 55
   fat loss principles 48
   frequency 49, 55
   hips 118–119
   incidental 98
   incorrect 12
   intensity 50–51, 56
   lower body 41
   mental state 33
   potbellies 124–128
   super fat loss 62
   thighs 112–117
   variety, if over thirty 51
   when sick 54

fat
   addiction 83
   burning 40
   rate of loss 36, 90
fats 80–86
females 34–5, 47
fibre 76
   causes fat loss 78
   health benefits 79
   insoluble 78
   soluble 78
   sources 79
fish 97
fitness
   measuring 53
food
   before bed 38
   low–fat 84–5, 99
   nutritious 76
   raw 76–7
   when to eat 95, 98
fruit 87, 90, 97

glycogen 22

habits 26
herbal teas 97
hips 118–119

iron 101

jogging 42, 55

kilojoules 79–80
   reducing intake 105–110

lunch 91, 102

margarine 84, 102
meat 84
menopause 35
mental attitude 25
metabolic rate
   slowing down 6
   speeding up 7
milkshakes, fruit 96
mineral water 97
mirror test 10
monosodium glutamate 13
muscle 43
muscle–stimulating exercise 40
muscle–toning exercise 124
myths about slimming 16–17

natural appetite reduction 99
natural low–energy sweetener 104
nutritional program 91
nutritious food 76

obesity 37
overeating 89–90
overexercise 54
overweight body
   effects of 10–11
   how to tell 10

pinch test 10
popcorn 97
potbelly 37, 120–128
potatoes 96, 101
   recipes 155
pregnancy 34
processed foods 13–15
pulse
   maximum rate 52
   measurement 53

raw food 76–7
recreation 30
reinforcement techniques 27, 31–2
relapses 33
rowing machine 61

salad recipes 147
self–monitoring 27
sit-ups 59
skipping 57
smoking 123
snacks 87–9, 102
soup recipes 144
stimulus control 26
stress release 28–31
sugar 80–81
   cravings 45
   reducing intake 86
super fat-loss exercises 62
swimming 55

target heart rate 52
thighs 112–117

vegetables 97
   recipes 131
vitamins 100

waistline fat 120
waist-to-hip ratio 10
walking 42, 55
water-drinking 53, 99
water retention 98
weight control
   common questions 36–8
weight loss
   plateaux 85–6
   preparations 38

yo-yo dieting 21